Raw Food Recipes

BETTER HEALTH, MORE ENERGY,

Freedom from Chronic Illness

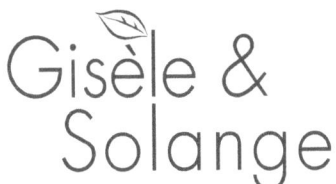

Gisèle &
Solange

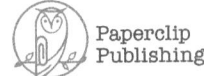
Paperclip
Publishing

RAW FOOD RECIPES: BETTER HEALTH, MORE ENERGY, AND FREEDOM FROM CHRONIC ILLNESS

Copyright © 2025 by Gisèle and Solange Adechian

Published by: Paperclip Publishing LLC

Editor: Nathan Miller

Cover & Interior Design: Diane M. Serpa

Library of Congress Control Number: 2024943758

ISBN: 979-8-9891077-4-2 (paperback)

ISBN: 979-8-9891077-5-9 (hardcover)

ISBN: 979-8-9891077-6-6 (eBook)

Printed by IngramSpark in the United States of America

First Printing: 2025

Paperclip Publishing LLC

3800 W Ray Road Suite 5

Chandler, AZ 85226

www.paperclippublishing.com

Special Thanks

To our parents

We want to thank our parents, Mrs. Assany Karamatou & Mr. Adechian Michel, for the love, knowledge, kindness and support given to us all our years as we grew up. We were children who grew up on different continents and experienced different cultures, which makes us who we are today as adults and grants us the ability to better navigate health challenges.

Special gratitude to our Mother for her patience and wisdom in finding the right balance between her work and raising us in the best possible way she could. Part of our inspiration for this book came from our roots, and especially our mother.

To our children (the next generation): We thank our children for allowing us to grow in health knowledge and experience through their own wellness journey.

CONTENTS

The Authors

Solange Adechian, Doctor in Life Sciences & Health, specialist of Nutrition, Naturotherapist, Coach in Yoga & Meditation.

Born from adventurous parents, Solange traveled through several countries in Africa, Europe, and Asia during her childhood. While in Africa, in Benin, she first developed ocular and visual migraines at the age of 8. These became more and more painful as she grew up.

In 1996 she relocated to Beijing (China), where her parents worked. Solange endured a number of medical tests that concluded there was nothing abnormal with her. However, her ocular and visual migraines were persistent and difficult to endure. She started to do a lot of research in order to understand the origin of her migraines and explored the impact of food and environment on her health.

Living in the midst of a traditional Chinese culture as a teen, Solange quickly became fascinated by traditional Chinese medicine. More importantly, she was struck by the impact of nutrition and the quality of food on the health of the Chinese people. She carefully observed the food, environment and physical activities of the Chinese people. Upon her return from China, she decided to settle in France where she began studying Biology and Nutrition.

Solange Adechian, PhD, has published scientific reviews in Nutrition & Health. She started her nutrition career working on clinical studies at the Agricultural Research and Human Nutrition Laboratory, Clermont-Ferrand-Theix in France. She wanted to understand the impact of

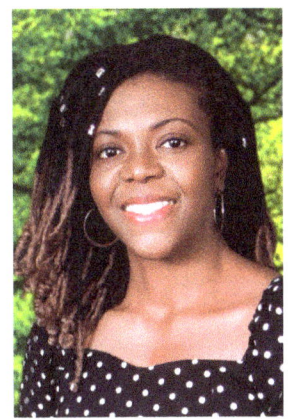

a protein-rich diet on weight loss in overweight and elderly people and the effect it has on inflammatory diseases of these people.

Solange helped many people–adults and children–who reduced their body fat weight while maintaining their bone mass and good health throughout the weight loss process.

She believes that a good diet, rich in protein, can improve muscle mass in elderly or people suffering from inflammatory diseases. She has dedicated her life working to understand the impact of nutrition and food quality in people's lives along with their ability to ingest and eliminate food.

After her doctorate, Solange decided she wanted to continue the adventure initiated by her parents and settled in Montreal (Canada). After going through dietary changes, paying attention to food quality, and despite all her knowledge acquired in nutrition, Solange was still confronted with health problems. While she had made progress treating her migraines back in France, these issues worsened once in Canada, followed by obesity and chronic diseases.

After substantial research, medical tests and endless drug treatments – not to mention the side effects – Solange decided to take back control of her health by engaging in allopathic medicine as an alternative path to healing.

Throughout all her experiences, Solange quickly understood that nutrition alone was not enough to improve our health. Thus, nutrition should be an integrative component of a holistic lifestyle.

She had a passionate desire to know and treat the cause of her illnesses rather than focus on the consequences each time. It was then she decided to resume studies that would eventually call into question all her knowledge acquired during her time at the university. After participating in a conference in Germany focusing on the links between chronic diseases, the digestive system and the liver, she began to study Naturopathy & Naturotherapy, yoga and meditation.

Today, Solange is completely cured of all her illnesses. In order to help all those who are going through similar health challenges, but above all to prevent people from going through the same issues, Solange joined with her sister, Gisèle, in creating a wellness company. Their mission is to help and empower people to understand the benefits of prevention and natural medicine on their health through holistic approaches, considering the integration of the body, mind and soul.

Gisèle Adechian, MBA, Raw Food Chef Plant-Based, Certified Integrative Nutrition Health Coach.

Gisèle started her career as a certified Lean Six Sigma Green Belt Project Manager and later as a Scrum Master, working for international companies and helping them understand the root causes of defects in their operational processes. Like Solange, she was born in Africa (Gabon) and raised in China (Beijing). Later she moved to France, where she received her MBA and two other master degrees: one in Communication and the other in Science, Quality of Health from the prestigious University of Compiègne.

Not long after relocating to New York (USA) in 2013, Gisèle started going through some health challenges. A year later she was diagnosed with asthma. After giving birth to her daughter in 2014, things did not get better. Gisèle realized that, though she was successful after accumulating a decade's worth of experience in project management, her health was still not optimal.

Her health started deteriorating as she went from one emergency room to another for about 4 years. Her life was changed in December, 2018 when she visited her sister in Canada. Gisèle almost lost her life during that trip as she struggled to breathe one day. If not for some holistic approaches to healing used by her sister Solange, she may not have survived!

Upon her return to the U.S., as if the universe wanted to make it clear to her that she needed to change her course

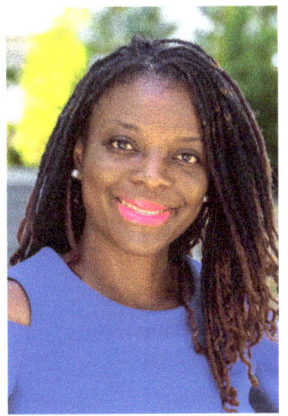

of action to improve her health, her daughter's allergies turned severe. This prompted her to make a life-changing decision on January 13, 2019: She decided to adopt a raw plant-based lifestyle.

Gisèle started researching courses online to eat well and go raw. She landed a raw certification course that led her to become a Raw chef. From there, she reversed her asthma in 10 months and improved her daughter's allergies by making lifestyle changes and using food as medicine.

Not until after her divorce did Gisèle realize that wellness is much more than food. Gisèle went on to become a Certified Integrative Nutrition Health Coach as a way to incorporate the Mind and Soul approaches to the Body nourishment knowledge she already had.

Today, she is on a mission to help other women prevent or heal themselves from auto-immune diseases using holistic approaches to wellness. She is also cofounder of their wellness company with her sister. Together, they decided to take their story to the world and empower others.

Preface

Dr. L. Scholosser, who worked on the ancient art of healing, said, "Life is sacred and its greatest virtue is health."

Each disease has double origins: One is psychological (mental) through negative thoughts. The other is related to unhealthy food choices, which may result in a digestive saturation that disturbs the elimination process. This, in turn, may involve an increase in the metabolic residuals and a clogging of blood, lymph and lacunar fluids.

Dr. Jauvais, in his book, *What to Eat to be Healthy, Slim and Stay Young*, explains the impact of psychology and bromatology on our health. We believe that each of us can live happily, healthy, in peace, in joy and in harmony with nature. Each person is capable of taking control over their overall well-being and health. It is in this context that the recipes in this book have been created. We hope to bring you happiness and well-being through raw, varied, simple and living recipes.

Through the recipes in this book, you will learn about the art and secret of living simply, while remaining young, beautiful, slim and healthy. The authors of this cookbook, Solange and Gisèle Adechian, are both passionate about nature and using food as medicine. They are also great adventurers who have traveled four continents of the world (Africa, Asia, North America and Europe). Both are full of enriching experiences. Here, they share some of them with you.

From their widely varied experiences, they've discovered that nutrition should be applied in a holistic, integrative, specific way and not simply as "mundane nutrition" focused solely on food. Well-being comes first and foremost from the pleasure of eating well—that is to say proper, adequate, natural, raw, and living food.

In this guide, you may be surprised to discover new things and to learn more about spices that heal. It is important to remain open-minded and do your own experiments based on some of our recommendations. That way you can assess the positive effects on your health. Perhaps it's time to let go of ancient ideas that often hinder our explorations of new avenues to natural health through new recipes.

I preserve my health:

The link between food and health has been documented since ancient times. Illness is the result of a decrease in the vital force—a sign of alarm from the body crying out for help—as a result of poor nutrition and accumulated negative thoughts.

Thus we understand very clearly that if the father of any disease is a negative thought, the mother is inappropriate nourishment. This is often misunderstood.

The famous quote from Hippocrates, "Let food be thy medicine," is mentioned in many papers. We still need to know what type of food it is, its nature, its specificity and its assimilation in the body to keep us healthy.

A poor diet, that is to say an unsuitable diet (carnivorism, extreme veganism, etc.), cooked or completely denatured, is part of the root causes of diseases. In the 19th century, the chemist and biologist Louis Pasteur once said "The germ is nothing. The terrain is everything," which suggests that any disease is curable if the body maintains all its potential to purify and clean itself properly on its own. We have to give it the necessary means to achieve such a mission.

A natural, raw, specific, adapted, living diet provides us with a good internal, vital, deep hygiene that keeps our electromagnetic field balanced and connects us to our spirituality and our internal God, which some naturopathic doctors call "the universal intelligence."

The body needs to be cleaned, not only externally, but also internally. It is by providing our body with "living" raw fruits and vegetables, micro-sprouts and fermented foods that we allow it not only to clean itself but also to revitalize itself in depth. As humans evolved and discovered fire, their food choices became dramatically more diversified and expanded. However, access to a wide variety of foods and the discovery of different methods of preparation does not mean that all foods are good for our health.

Breast milk is a uniquely complete food. It provides all the nutrients that human beings need for growth. However, after breastfeeding we no longer need any milk to supply nutrition. Instead, we can use a wide variety of milk substitutes. In the event an animal-based milk is absolutely necessary, one may choose goat milk, for example, since it is scientifically proven that goat milk is closer to human milk.

Anatomo-physiological scientific studies clearly show that, biologically, the digestive tract of humans is very similar to that of the great apes—whether we admit it or not. So our evolutionary origins would call for a diet that looks more like this:

- Fruitarian: 40% fresh, raw fruits and 20% dried sweetened fruits;
- Vegan: 20% vegetables;
- Carnivore: 10% raw seafood, raw egg yolks or raw fish, 5% raw meat;
- Starch: 5% sweet starch (potatoes, etc.)

Please note that in North America, most of the fruits are acidic because they are imported.

The digestion of food begins in the mouth and ends in the anus (a tract that is, on average, 9 meters in total). Many scientific studies have shown the important health benefits of chewing. It is important to take the time to eat well, without being stressed—preferably in a quiet and peaceful place. Poor digestion can impact our immune system because immune cells lie in the gut. "All diseases begin in the intestine," according to a principle of Hippocrates.

According to food combining theory, foods that are not complementary can cause indigestion, gas, acidity and the formation of toxins. However, when eaten separately, the same foods can support proper digestion.

Herbert M. Shelton, Doctor of Naturopathic Medicine, was one of the first food combination initiators in the 1900s. When a food is not well assimilated, people can suffer from annoying symptoms like indigestion or other health disorders. Thus, the digestion of proteins requires an acid environment while the digestion of carbohydrates requires an alkaline environment. Digestive disorders and constipation may be signs of a bad food combination and poor nutrient absorption.

By consuming protein-rich foods (poultry, fish, etc.) along with foods rich in carbohydrates (bread, rice, etc.), the food environment becomes neutral, which adversely affects digestion. Note: Food combination is based on observational studies rather than scientifically proven. Despite the fact that nowadays it is difficult to find food combination philosophy in scientific literature, awareness of food combination can serve as a guideline for improving health, such as weight loss, skin health, gut health and particularly digestion.

Dr. Gundry wrote in his book, "What you stop eating has a much greater impact on our health than what you start eating." (Dr. Gundry talks in detail about this in his book, *The Hidden Dangers of Healthy Eating*).

It has been observed that a simple water-based fasting can cure certain diseases. It is essential that the patient seeks medical pre- and post-consultation with a physician. You will realize that if you pamper your intestine by providing it with the foods it needs, not only will your liver do well but your intestines will too. Indeed, the liver is the second largest organ of our body (after the skin) and the largest gland of the body. The liver alone performs more than 500 functions.

If you want to live a long, young and healthy life, this may be the time to take control of your health and stand up for yourself. Give priority to raw foods, which are whole, living foods and transfer energy to us. Indeed, cooking at extreme temperatures kills the nutrients and enzymes in the food. This devitalizes the body and often makes people feel tired and sick. During the transition period to healing a chronic illness naturally, you can opt for gentle steamed cooking, with temperatures not exceeding 46°C (115°F). This prevents the food from becoming too denatured, preserving all the good nutrients. We are fortunate that the human body is endowed with an extraordinary intelligence. It adapts amazingly well to the various situations that are offered to it. There is a healthy congruence when the body is fed with foods that are natural and adapted to its growth.

When we talk about healthy, natural, raw and living foods, we are talking about raw, uncooked foods, or foods cooked at a temperature below 37°C (98.6°F). This includes sprouts, algae, fresh vegetables and raw proteins. *Note: Living food gives life! Unlike a raw egg, a cooked chicken egg will not yield a chick!*

Here's what your day should look like in general:

1. Start the morning with meditation. This is a great way to show gratitude to mother nature for a new day and for being alive. Be happy for your health or embrace where you are in your healing journey. You can also do short stretching exercises and/or Yoga.

2. Get into the habit of tongue scraping to prevent bacteria from building up in your mouth and to prevent bad breath. Drink a glass of warm water to rinse your organs after the long work they have undertaken overnight while you were asleep.

3. Have breakfast consisting of raw and living foods (fresh and juicy fruits, dried fruits, compote or prepared fresh fruit salad, and vegetable milk). You can choose a recipe from the many suggestions in this book. You have in this book a variety of recipes ranging from fresh juices, smoothies, fruit salads and nuts, nut milk, etc. While eating, be mindful of the way you chew your food and salivate well.

4. At noon, have lunch. We offer some top picks in this book. Ideally, start your meal with a nutritious juice as a starter (e.g., a raw juice obtained from adding fruits and/or vegetables to a juice extractor). We suggest using a juice extractor,

which maximizes the juice to pulp ratio (more juice and less pulp). This is based on the rewarding experiences we have had using several juice extractors on the market. If you don't have one, you can also use a high-speed blender and a nut milk bag to extract the juice. Your lunch can either be a salad made with raw and/or fermented vegetables, or consist of a large bowl of fruits.

Soups are taken last, after juices and meals. Do not eat sweet desserts right after a savory meal because the enzymes that facilitate the digestion of a sweet meal are different from those of a savory meal.

Also, do not mix fruits and protein during the same meal.

5. Take a relaxing herbal tea between meals. Examples of teas that help the liver include boldo, dandelion, milk thistle and artichoke. Hot peppermint tea aids with digestion. You might also consider taking verbena tea to relax.

6. Have a dinner made up of the various recipes that we offer in this guide.

7. At the end of the meal, it is recommended to go for a walk to facilitate the digestion process. As a Chinese proverb says: "100 steps after each meal brings you closer to 100 years old." Keep in mind that contrary to what most people think, a fruit is not a dessert, and should be considered like a meal. One mission of this book is to provide you with the necessary knowledge you need to be the master of your body, your health and your well-being.

8. Before going to bed, practice a relaxation activity such as Tai Chi or meditation. Then make yourself a foot bath with warm water and ginger or Guérande salt. We are happy to share our wonderful daily routine and experience with you. For any consultation in Naturopathy or requests for Holistic Nutrition Health Coaching, visit our website https://www.wellnessauthors.com/

All the recipes in this book should be made with natural, organic and raw Ingredients as much as possible. The recipes in this book are gluten-free, dairy-free and refined sugar-free. They have also been written with lots of passion, love and joy.

Please note: Many of our recipes call for use of a high-speed blender. You may think, "a blender is a blender." It basically comes down to the power of the machine. When making professional cakes or blending smoothly, we recommend a blender with a minimum of 1000-1500 watts of power. If you are able to get a high-speed blender, it will prove a worthy investment!

A note about ingredient substitutions: Some Ingredients are seasonal and individual preferences vary for several reasons (e.g. allergies). Here is a list of substitutions that may be made:

List of substitutions

INGREDIENTS	SUBSTITUTIONS
Almond	Coconut, tiger nuts
Almond milk	Coconut milk, tiger nut milk
Coconut nectar	Agave nectar
Macadamia nuts	Brazil nuts, cashews
Turmeric	Ginger
Kale	Spinach
Cucumber	Zucchini
Baobab	Soursop
Pomegranate	Passion fruit
Mango	Pineapple or any other fruit containing water
Pineberries	Strawberries
Almond butter	Tahini
Lakanto monkfruit sweetener	Mesquite powder or simply omit
Pumpkin seeds	Any other seeds or nuts

Make it Nut-Free

These recipes from the cookbook do not contain nuts so can be appropriate for people with nut allergies or if you simply prefer to explore something else than nuts.

- Ceylon Hibiscus Juice With Cinnamon
- Turmeric Infusion
- Clove & Tamarind Juice
- Raw Beet Juice With Fresh Ginger
- Green Anise & Rosemary Infusions
- Carrots, Beets & Kale Juice
- Kale, Apples, & Black Radish Juice
- Pineapple, Mango & Kefir Juice
- Carrots, Parsley & Black Radish Juice
- Kale & Beet Juice Coodles
- Summer Salad
  (*excluding the dressing*)

- Cucumber Roll
  (*excluding the dressing*)
- Raw Tacos
  (*excluding the raw cheese*)
- Thyme Seasoning
- Basil Tomato Sauce
- Exotic Mangosteen & Dragon Fruit Salad
- Pineapple Cherry Delish
  (*replace almonds with tiger nuts*)
- Apple Spinach Mix
  (*replace almonds with tiger nuts*)
- Strawberry Smoothie
  (*replace almonds with tiger nuts*)
- Guava Nectar
- Pomegranate Nectar
- Baobab Nectar

- Coconut Berry Smoothie
  (*excluding the toppings*)
- Peach Strawberry Smoothie
  (*replace almond milk with tiger nut milk*)
- Macaron Crust
- Macaron Filling
  (*from the Hibiscus Macaron Cheesecake recipe*)
- Pineapple Jelly
- Strawberry Frozen Ice Cream
- Raspberry Filling
  (*from the Raw Coconut Bar recipe*)
- Herbal Teas
- Poached Pear
  (*excluding the candied nuts*)

Disclaimers

In no way does this book intend to provide or replace medical advice.

The narrated stories and advice are solely based on our personal experiences.

Recipes with this sign contain Ingredients that can be easily sourced from West Africa.

The serving sizes given in this book are based on our personal recommendations and are in no way based on any regulations. Regulatory serving sizes may vary from country to country.

References

The Many Meanings of Food Combining, Dr.Deanna Minich; Oct 14, 2021, Medically Reviewed By, Jillian Kubala, MS, RD, Oct 13, 2021, written by Taylor Jones, edited by Cheryl S. Grant, Copy Edited by Jill Campbell, © 2023 Healthline Media LLC.

Les combinaisons alimentaires et votre santé : Pour bien digérer, les menus dissociés à la portée de tous, Herbert-M. Shelton, Editions de la nouvelle hygiène / Le courrier du livre, 3 janvier 1994, 126 p. (ISBN 978-2-7029-0055-0, lire en ligne [archive]).

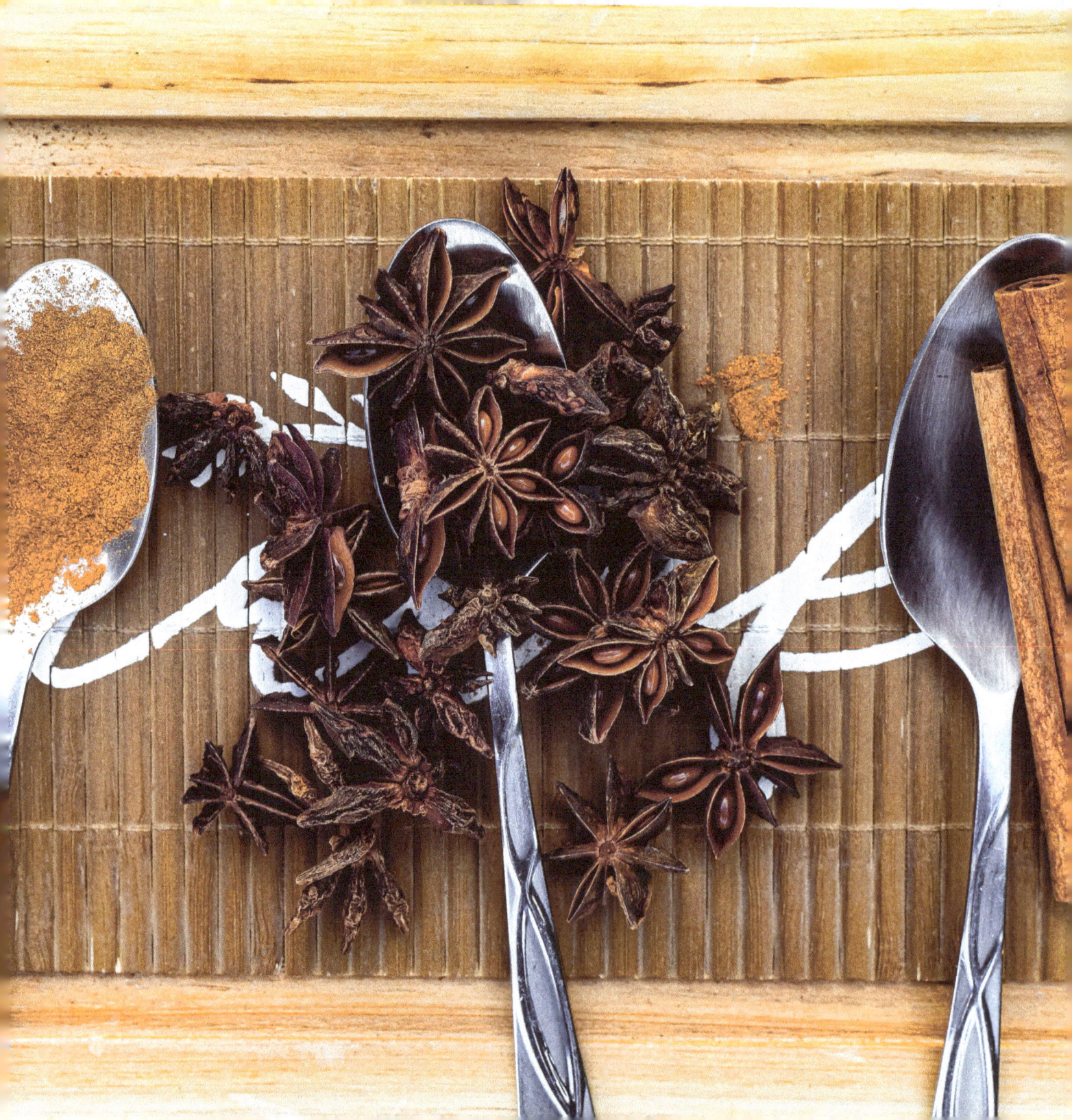

I
INFUSIONS & JUICES WITH HEALING SPICES

The power of spices that heal.

Spices, when used wisely, have healing powers.

Do not hesitate to put them regularly in your meals.

Or drink them like infusions or juices throughout the day!

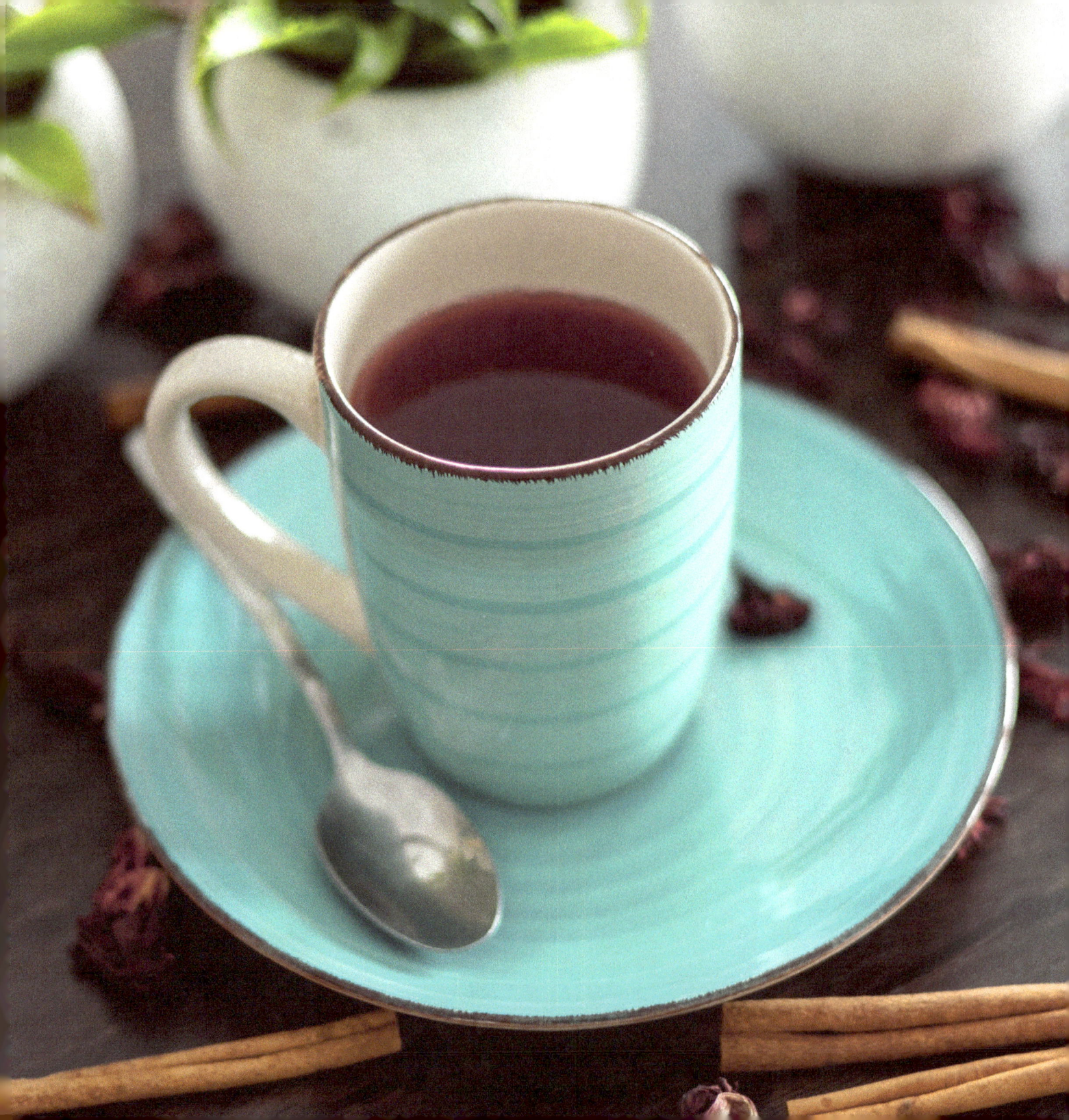

Ceylon's cinnamon Hibiscus Juice

Serving size: 1

Equipment
- Glass jar with lid
- Spoon
- Saucepan for boiling

Ingredients
- ½ Tbsp hibiscus flowers
- ½ stick Ceylon cinnamon
- 2 cups water

  +
- Juice of ½ lemon
- 3 Tbsp Coconut nectar

Instructions
1. Place hibiscus flowers, cinnamon stick and water in a pan. Boil for 5 minutes.
2. Remove from stove.
3. Filter to obtain hibiscus juice.
4. Let sit for 10 minutes.
5. Add lemon juice and coconut nectar to the filtered hibiscus juice. Stir well with a spoon.
6. Refrigerate or drink right away.

DID YOU KNOW? *Ceylon's Cinnamon*

Ceylon's cinnamon (*Cinnamomum Zeylanicum*), from Sri Lanka, is the bark of a tree called the cinnamon tree.

Cinnamon has many properties:

» Antiseptic

» Antiviral: used to relieve respiratory and intestinal problems

» Deworming properties: helps eliminate intestinal parasites

» Expectorant: helps relieve cough and lung bronchial conditions cardiotonic

» Astringent: helps to tighten the tissues

» Decongestant

» Anti-spasmodic: helps digestion and fights bloating. It also relieves abdominal cramps and colic.

» Stimulant: helps fight against fatigue

Be careful when purchasing cinnamon as some are counterfeit cinnamons from China or Burma, which contain a significant amount of coumarin with Ceylon cinnamon. Coumarin is potentially toxic and may cause liver damage. The bark of Chinese cinnamon (*Cinnamomum cassia*) is thicker (2–3 mm), has a stronger, vanilla-like odor and is more difficult to break than Ceylon's cinnamon (about 1 mm). Ceylon's cinnamon is firmer, sweeter and more brittle—easily broken by hand. Ceylon cinnamon, which should be preferred, contains very little or no coumarin.

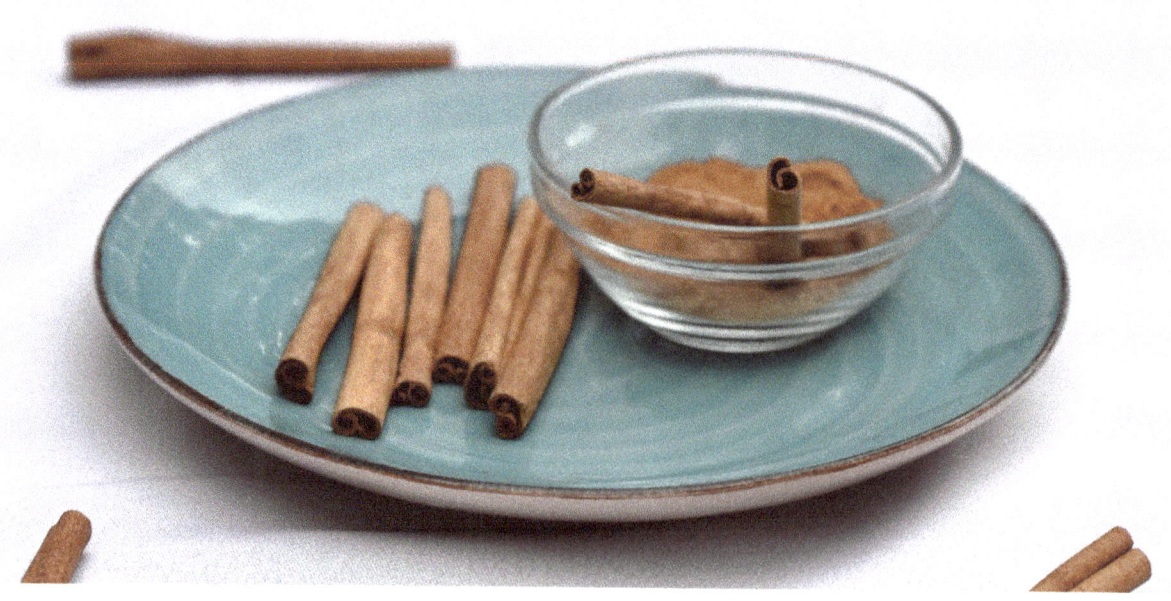

Treat Yourself
with Cinnamon

EXTINCTION OF VOICE:

Ingredients

- 1 cup hot water, filtered
- 1 tsp cinnamon powder
- 2 tsp honey

Instructions

Mix the hot water with cinnamon and honey. Drink immediately.

TONING THE HEART:

Ingredients

- Make a mixture of equal parts of:
  › honey
  › hawthorn or olive or lemon balm plants
  › cinnamon

Instructions

Drink in a little warm water every morning. (Hawthorn supports the heart muscle. The olive tree lowers tension. Lemon balm regulates the rhythm.)

NAUSEA:

Ingredients

- 1 tsp cinnamon powder
- 1 cup warm water

Instructions

Add cinnamon powder t,o warm water and drink. Repeat several times as needed.

FLU:

Ingredients

- ½ tsp cinnamon powder
- 3 whole cloves
  +
- 2 small eucalyptus plant leaves
- 2 small thyme leaves
  +
- juice of ½ lemon
- 2 tsp honey

Instructions

1. Boil cinnamon and cloves in one cup of water for 5 minutes.
2. Remove from stove and add eucalyptus and thyme leaves. Let steep for 2–5 minutes.
3. Filter and add lemon and honey.
4. Drink immediately.

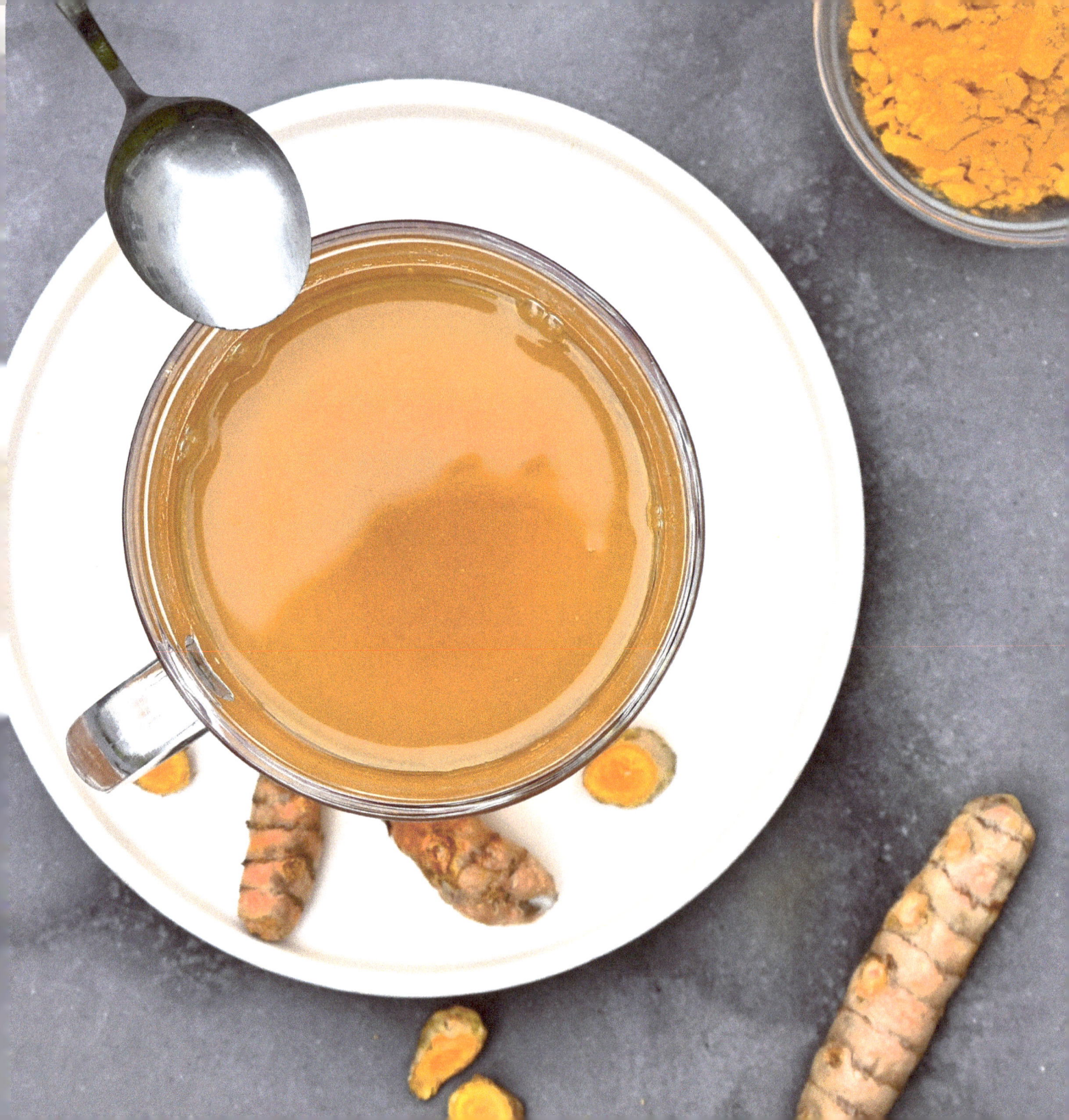

Turmeric Infusion

Serving size: 1

Equipment

- Pot
- Sieve
- Tea cup

Ingredients

- one 2-inch nub fresh turmeric (no need to peel)
- 2 cups water

  +
- 1 Tbsp honey or coconut nectar
- 1 tsp cinnamon powder

Instructions

1. To prepare turmeric, slice it into thin rounds (no wider than ¼-inch). Combine with water.
2. Bring the mixture to a simmer, then reduce the heat to maintain a gentle simmer for 2 minutes.
3. Remove the pot from heat. Gently pour mixture through a sieve to separate the tea from the turmeric.
4. Pour the tea into a cup. Add the second set of ingredients (honey or coconut nectar) and cinnamon powder and mix together.
5. Drink immediately.

DID YOU KNOW? *Turmeric*

Turmeric (*Curcuma longa*) or "Indian saffron" is obtained by grinding the dried rhizome of a tropical plant of the ginger family, mainly from India and Indonesia.

Turmeric has many properties:

» Anti-inflammatory: Turmeric's rhizome is one of the best plants with anti-inflammatory properties. It will help the body fight against inflammation, which is a process of defense when the body is faced with internal or external aggression.

» Anti-cancer: contains antioxidants, slowing down the process of cell oxidation

» Antibacterial & Antiseptic: preventing infection and reducing microbes

» Diuretic: increases urinary secretion

» Cleansing properties: purifies the body, promoting the elimination of toxins and organic waste.

» Turmeric helps to make the blood fluid. It controls fever and also lowers cholesterol.

» Decongestant

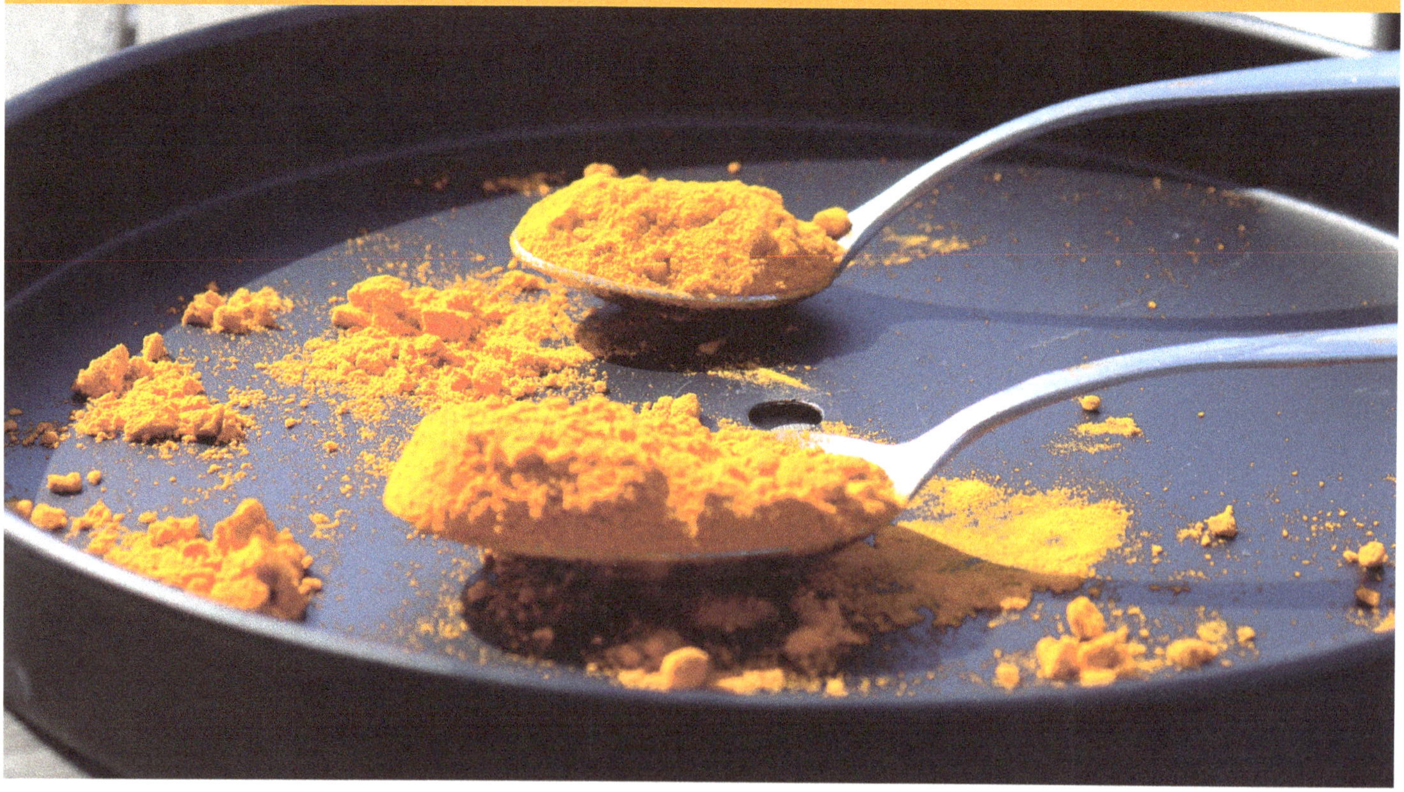

Treat Yourself
with Turmeric

DIARRHEA:

Ingredients
- 8 oz water, filtered
- 1 tsp turmeric powder

Instructions

Mix an 8 ounce glass of water with turmeric and drink.

ASTHMA:

Ingredients
- 1 cup almonds, soaked for 8 hours and dehydrated
- 3 cups water, filtered

  +
- 1 tsp turmeric, powdered
- honey *(optional)*

Instructions

1. Blend the almonds and the water in a high-speed blender until smooth.
2. Strain with a nut milk bag. *(Use only 1 cup of this milk for this recipe and store the remainder in refrigerator for future use.)*
3. Mix the powdered turmeric and the almond milk.
4. Drink 3 cups a day.
5. *Another option:* Mix an equal amount of honey and powdered turmeric and drink daily.

FLU:

Ingredients
- ½ tsp cinnamon powder
- 3 whole cloves

  +
- juice of ½ lemon
- 2 tsp honey
- 2 tsp turmeric powder
- 2 tsp cataria and fennel mixture

Instructions

1. Boil cinnamon powder and cloves for 5 minutes in a large cup of water.
2. Let remaining ingredients steep for 15 minutes.
3. Mix with first set of ingredients, filter and drink.

SKIN CONDITION:

Ingredients
- 1 tsp green clay
- 1 tsp Aloe Vera gel
- 1 tsp vegetable glycerin
- 1 tsp turmeric powder

Instructions

1. Make a poultice of ingredients.
2. Apply the above mixture to the skin.
3. Let it sit for 1 hour on your skin and rinse.

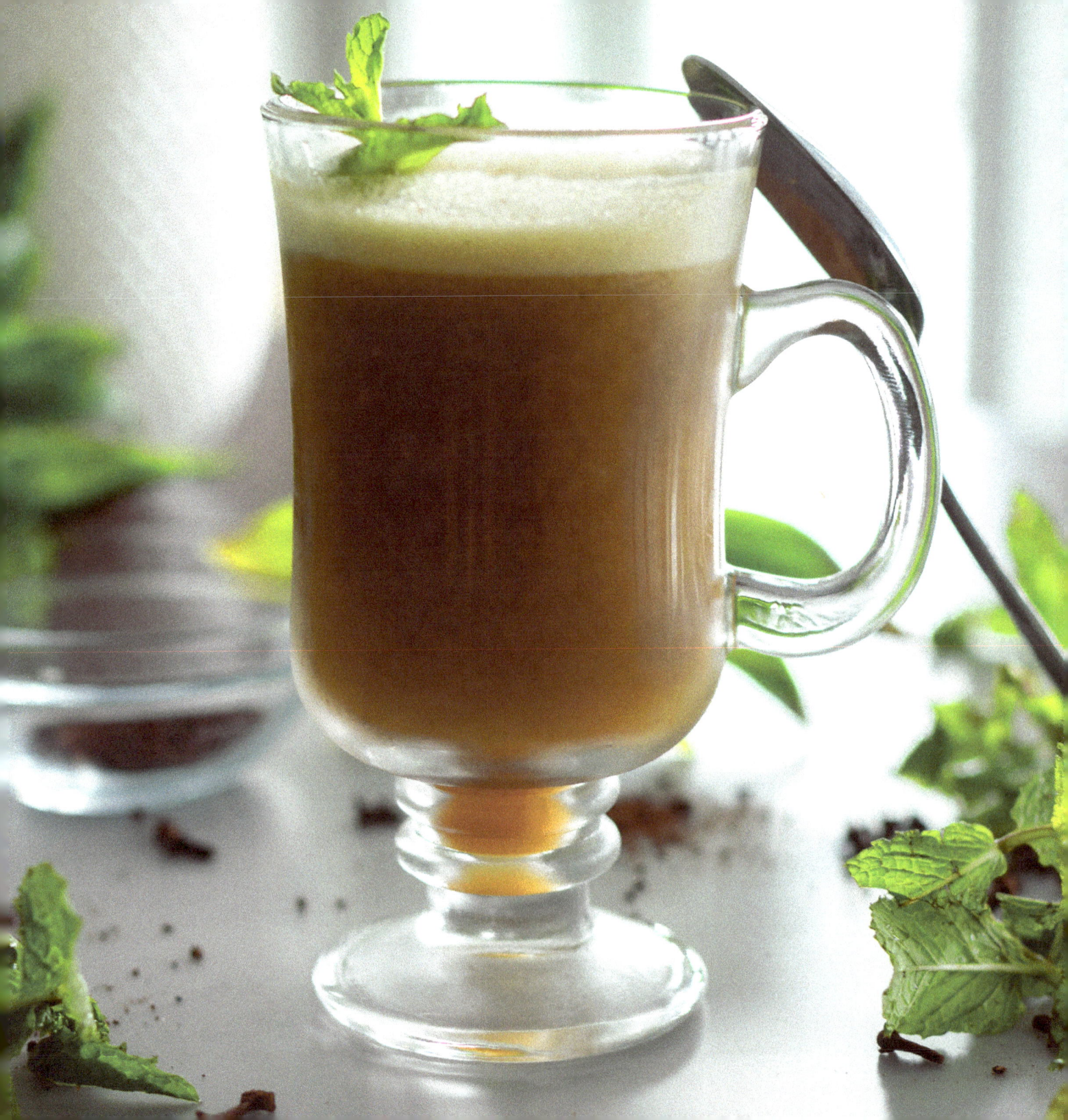

Clove & Tamarind Juice

Serving size: 1

Equipment
- Mason jar
- Wooden spoon
- High-speed blender

Ingredients
- 4 Tbsp tamarind, fresh
- 8 oz water

  +
- ½ tsp cloves, ground
- 2 fresh moringa leaves (or ½ tsp moringa powder)
- 4 soaked dates, pitted
- 4 mint leaves, fresh

Instructions
1. Soak the tamarind with 8 ounces of water in a glass for 24 hours. Set aside.
2. Blend the cloves, moringa, dates and mint leaves in a high-speed blender.
3. Add to water and tamarind mixture.
4. Filter, pour into mason jar and set aside in a cool place for at least 10 minutes before drinking.

DID YOU KNOW? *Clove*

Clove (*Syzygium aromaticum*) is an unborn bud of a clove tree that grows in tropical countries.

» Clove has many properties:

» Analgesic: Clove is very well known for calming dental pain.

» Antioxidant

» Anti-spasmodic

» Antiseptic, anti-infective and bactericidal

» Anti-rheumatic

» Expectorant: used in pulmonary conditions, asthma

» Deworming

» Digestive: for digestive and intestinal disorders, liver problems, colitis, neuralgia and intestinal parasites

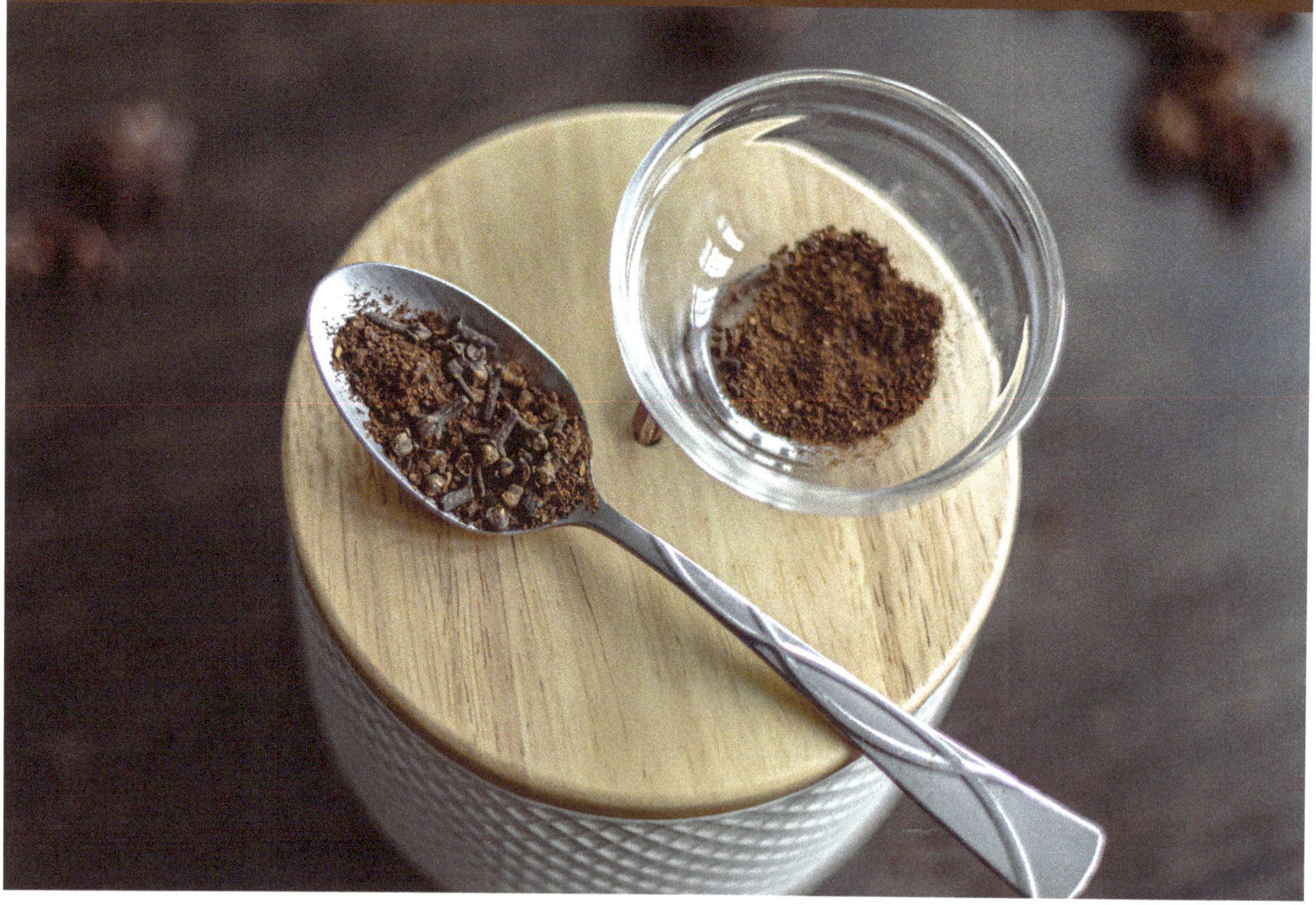

Treat Yourself
with Clove

TOOTHACHE:

Ingredients

1 or 2 whole cloves

Instructions

Chew one or two cloves and let them infuse on the hurting tooth.

ASTHMA:

Ingredients

- 1 cup water, filtered
- 10 whole cloves

Instructions

1. Boil water and cloves in a saucepan for about 5 minutes.
2. Filter and drink.

STOMACH PAIN:

Ingredients

5 or 6 whole cloves

Instructions

Suck on 5 or 6 cloves for a few minutes and discard.

FLU:

Ingredients

- ½ tsp cinnamon powder
- 3 whole cloves
- 1 cup water
  +
- juice of ½ lemon
- 2 tsp honey
- 2 tsp turmeric
- 2 tsp cataria leaves and fennel mixture

Instructions

1. Boil cinnamon and cloves in a cup of water for 5 minutes.
2. Let steep for 15 minutes.
3. Add second set of ingredients, then filter.
4. Drink immediately.

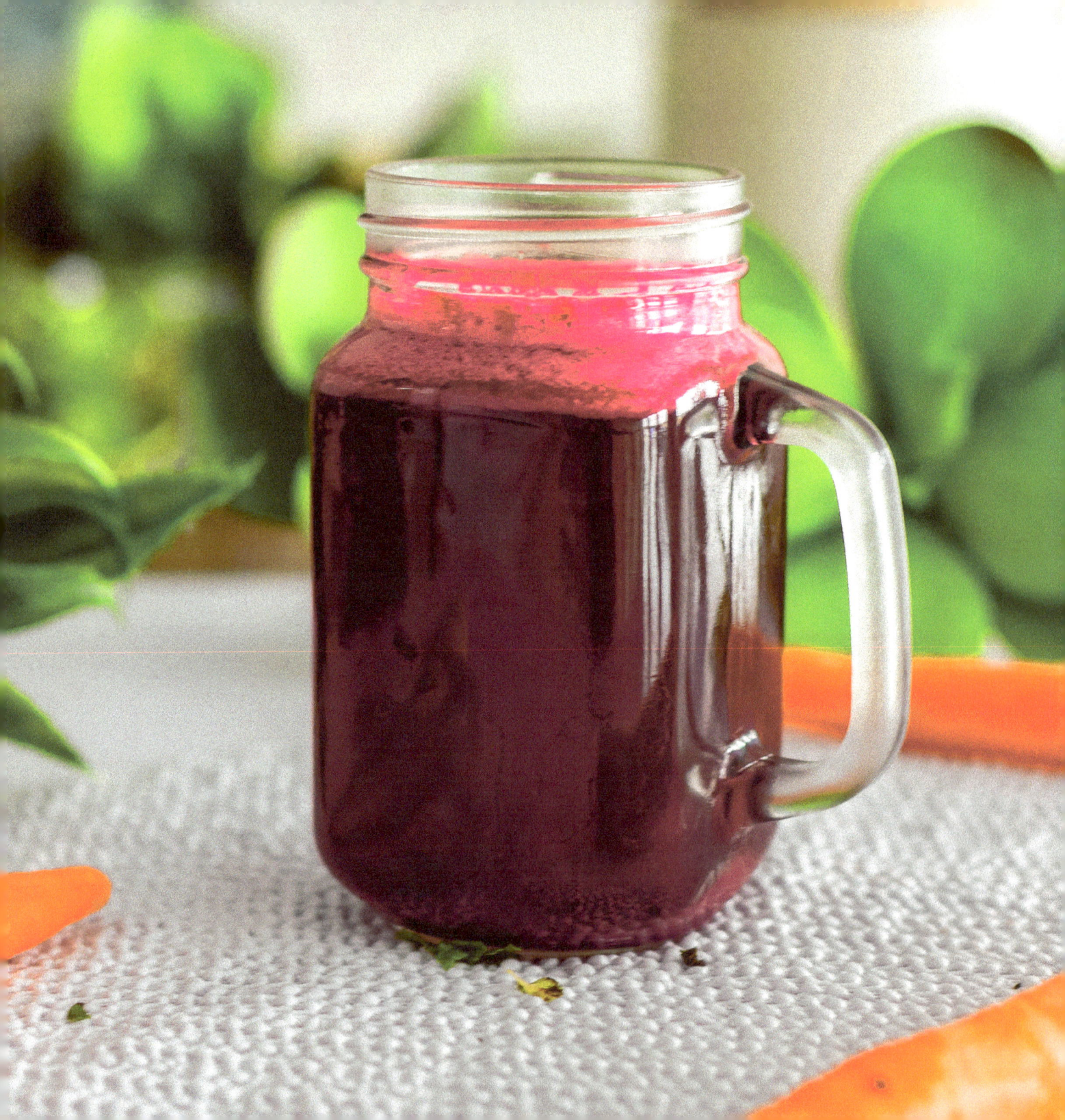

Raw Beet Juice with Fresh Ginger

Serving size: 1

Equipment

- Mason jar
- Spoon
- Juice extractor

Ingredients

- 2 fresh beets, raw
- 1 fresh apple
- 1 ginger root

Instructions

1. Extract the juice of beets, apple and ginger using a juice extractor. If you do not have a juice extractor, you can use a blender and filter with a nut milk bag *(Keep in mind that the taste might not be exactly the same as if you had a juice extractor)*.
2. If mixture is too thick, add water.
3. Drink immediately. Store in the refrigerator for up to 48 hours. *(Beyond 48 hours, the juice might lose its nutritional value and taste.)*

DID YOU KNOW? *Ginger*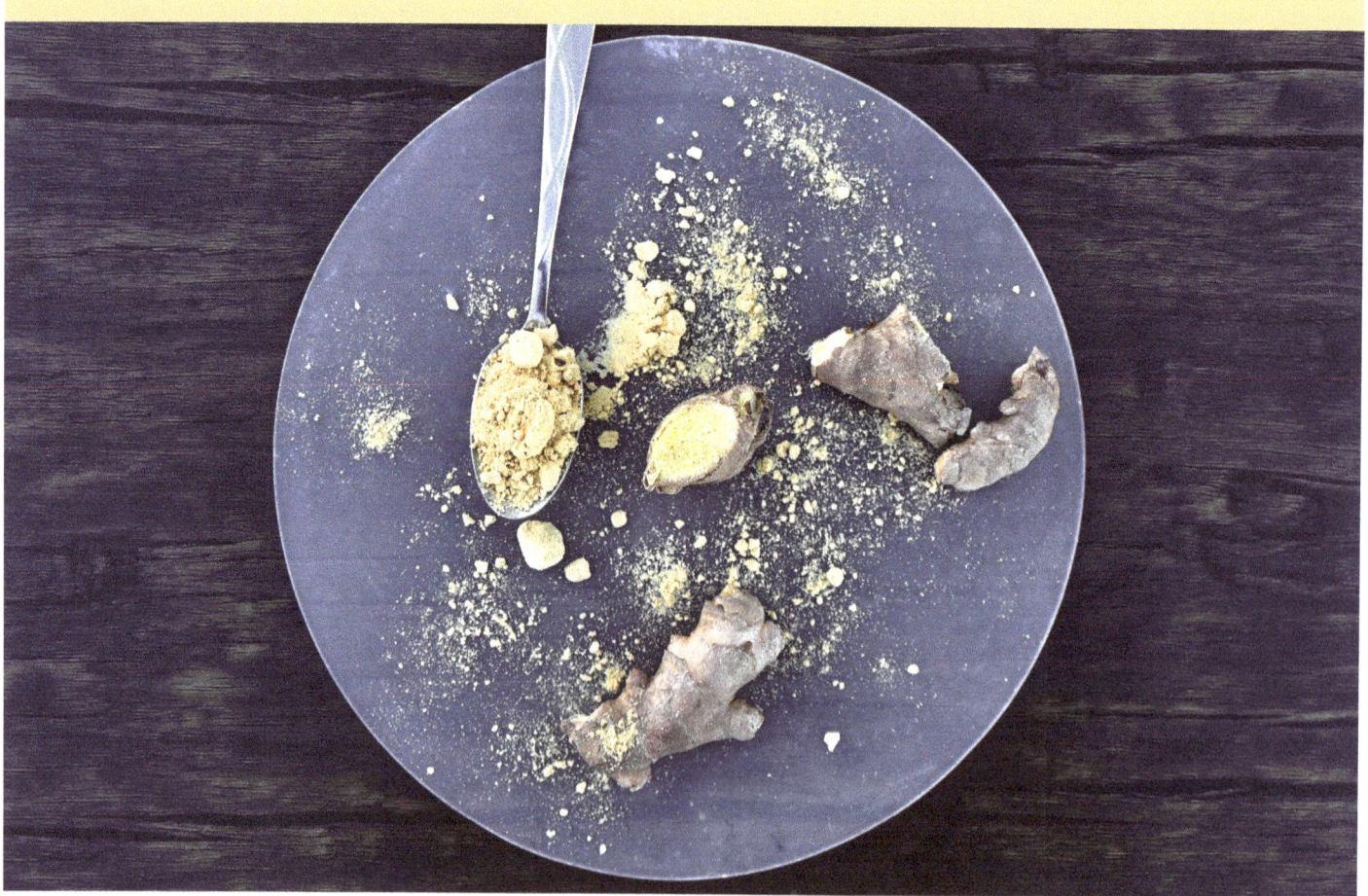

Ginger (*Zingiber officinale*) is a perennial herbaceous plant of the curcuma family. Ginger is widely used in most kitchens around the world.

» Ginger has many properties:

» Anti-nausea

» Antioxidant: It is involved in the prevention of cancer cells by blocking angiogenesis and stimulating the immune system.

» Antibacterial

» Antiseptic

» Digestive: One root of fresh grated ginger should be eaten during each meal for easy digestion.

» Analgesic

» Anti-migraine

» Expectorant: Thanks to its digestive properties, it protects the liver and facilitates the secretion of bile.

Treat Yourself

with Ginger

CONSTIPATION:

Ingredient

1 ginger root, fresh

Instruction

Consume (*chew*) 1 root of fresh grated ginger during each meal.

OSTEOARTHRITIS:

Ingredient

1 ginger root, fresh

Instruction

Make fresh ginger juice compresses to place on painful parts.

ASTHMA:

Ingredients

- 2 leaves thyme, fresh
- 2 cups water, filtered
  +
- 1 ginger root
- 1 tsp moringa or lobelia powder

Instructions

1. Make a thyme infusion and add the root of fresh ginger and moringa or lobelia.
2. Strain and drink immediately.

FLU / BRONCHITIS:

Ingredients

- ½ tsp cinnamon powder
- 3 whole cloves
- 8 oz water
  +
- juice of ½ lemon
- 1 root fresh ginger
- 3 tsp ginger leaf, powdered
- 1 tsp black pepper, ground
- 2 tsp honey
- 2 tsp turmeric, ground

Instructions

1. Boil a large cup of water for 5 minutes with cinnamon and cloves.
2. Let steep for 15 minutes, filter and add the second set of ingredients before drinking.

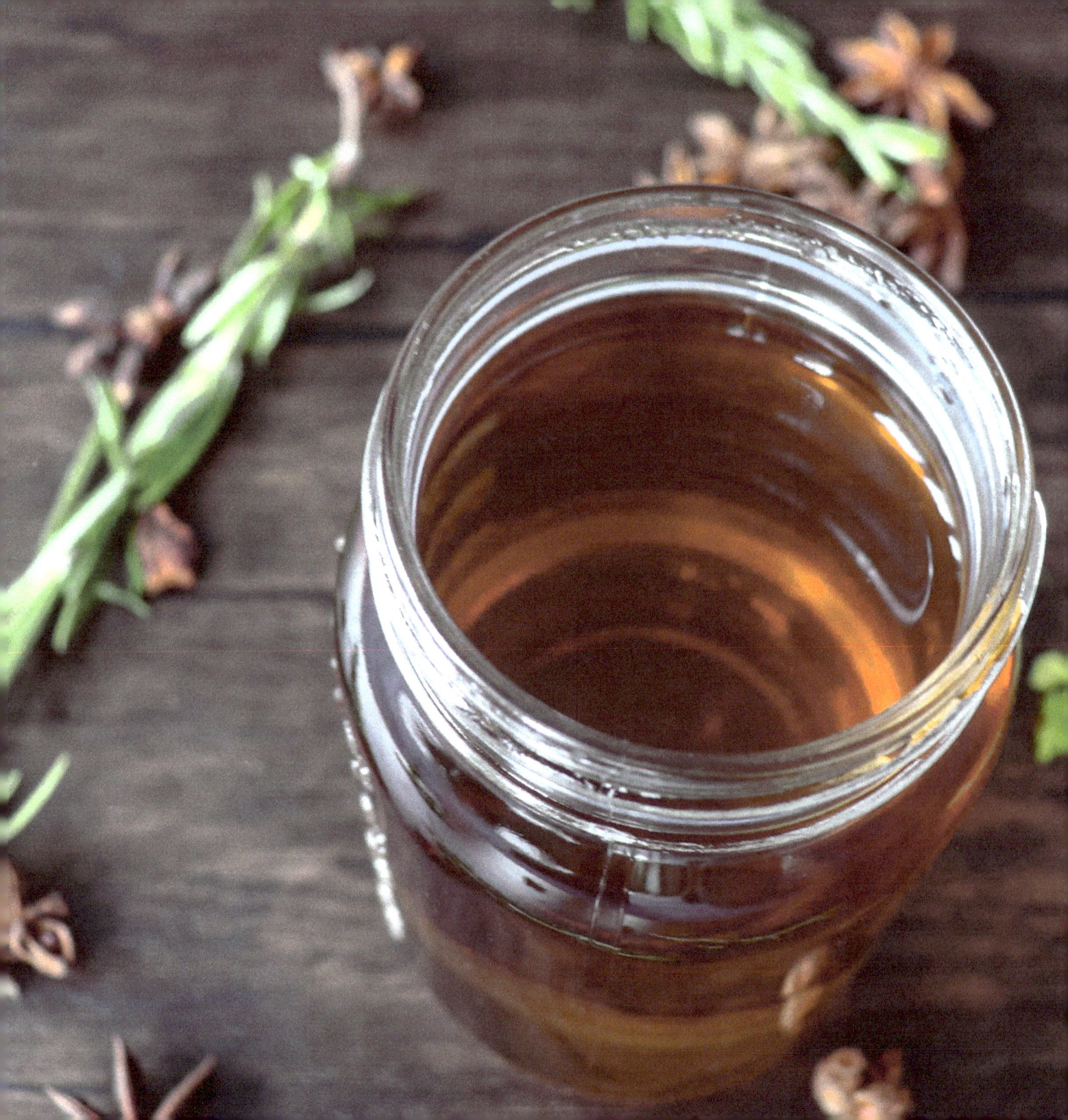

Star Anise & Rosemary Infusions

Serving size: 1

Equipment

- Cooking pan (to boil)
- Mason jar
- Spoon

Ingredients

- 1½ cups water, filtered
- 3 tsp dried star anise
- 1 tsp rosemary leaf, fresh

Instructions

1. Boil water with star anise and rosemary for 3 minutes.
2. Strain.
3. Let cool to 98.6°F (37°C).
4. Stir and pour into mason jar.

DID YOU KNOW? *Star Anise*

Star anise is usually used as a spice in food culture.

Star anise has many properties:

» Antioxidant

» Anti-inflammatory

» Gastroprotective: aids in food transit

» Expectorant

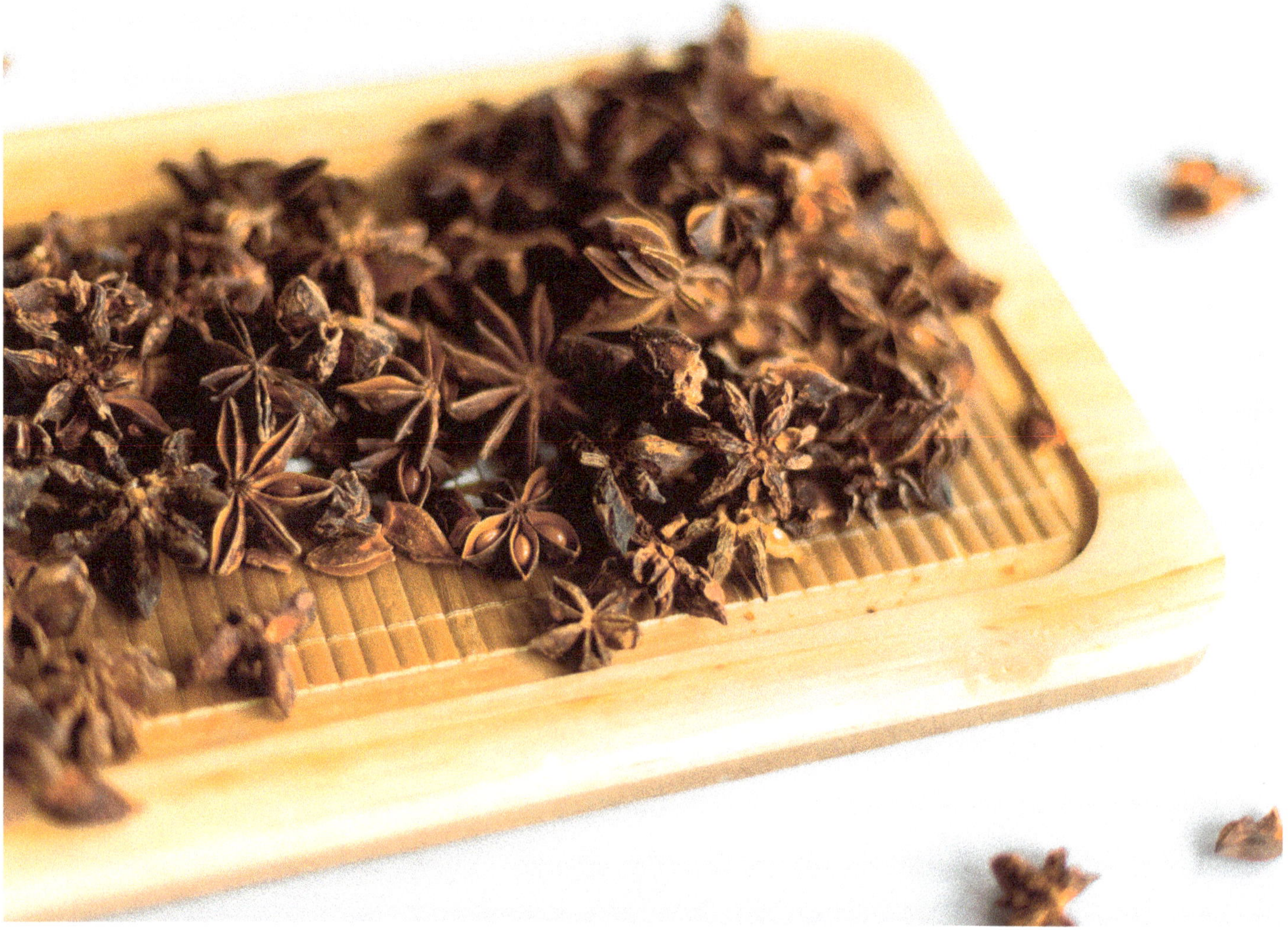

Treat Yourself
with Star Anise

TOOTHACHE:

Ingredients

    1–2 star anise seeds

Instructions

    Chew 1 or 2 star anise seeds and let it infuse on the hurting tooth.

COSMETICS:

Make your own lip balm, candle and soap with star anise. Simply email us through our website for details: **https://www.wellnessauthors.com/**.

References

"*Guide Hachette DES PLANTES MÉDICINALES,*" ISBN 978-2-01-238412-5, 2012

"*Croquez la Vie ! Des aliments qui guérissent et qui préviennent,*" Dr. Georges Pamplona-Roger, ISBN 978-84-7208-127-7, 2009

"*D'ici et d'ailleurs Les Epices qui guérissent,*" Murielle Toussaint, EAN 9782849391112, 2015

"*Nouveau style de vie Santé par les Aliments,*" Dr. Georges Pamplona-Roger, ISBN 978-84-7208-288-5, 2009

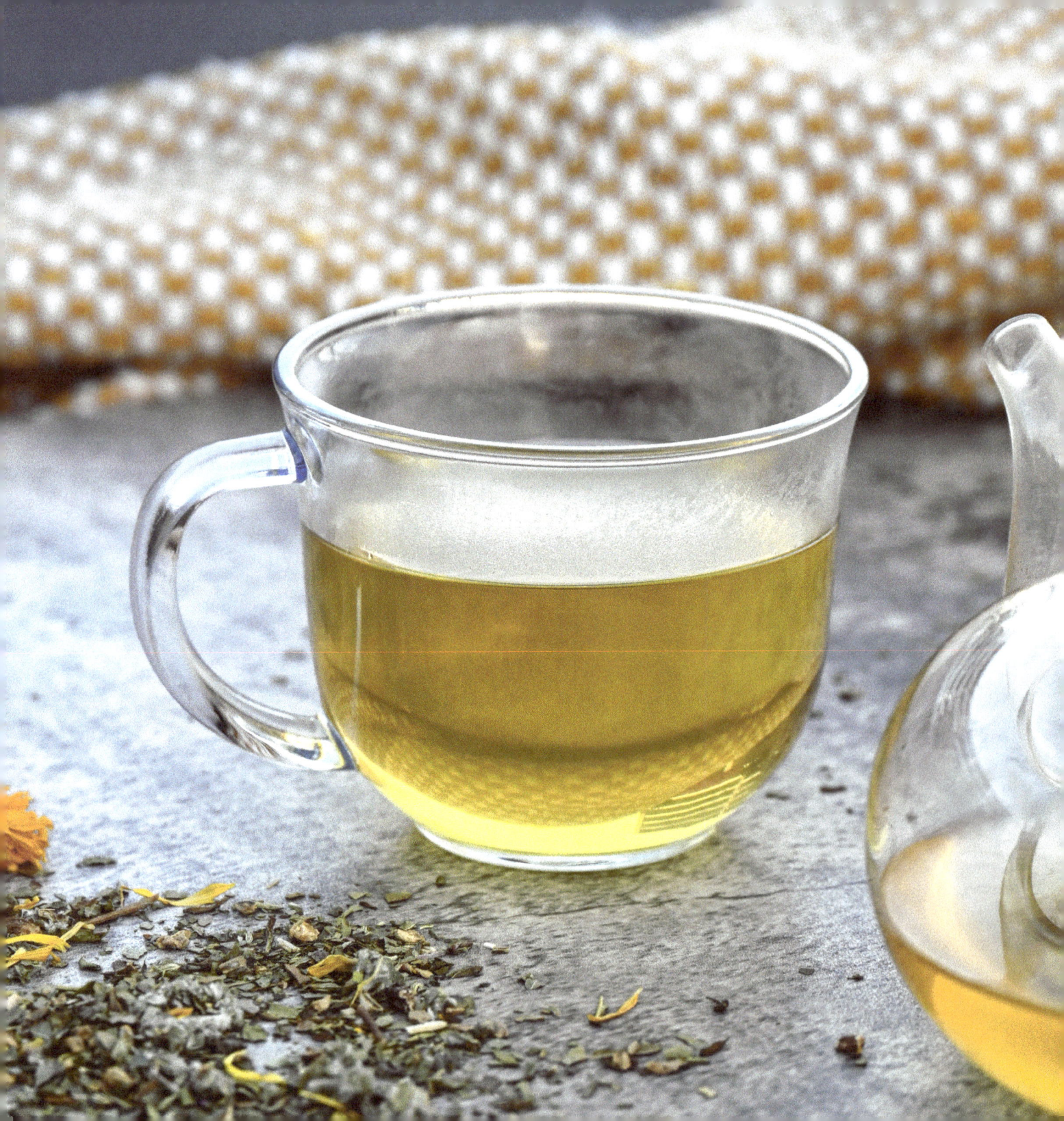

II
CURE WITH PLANTS

The Healing Power of Plants

Plants are powerful when you know which one to use and how to combine them. They can be a great way to support our health and uu boost our immune system.

Liver Plus
Detox Formula

Cold Formula

Stress Formula 1

Immune
System Boost

Stress Formula 2

Kidney
Detox Formula

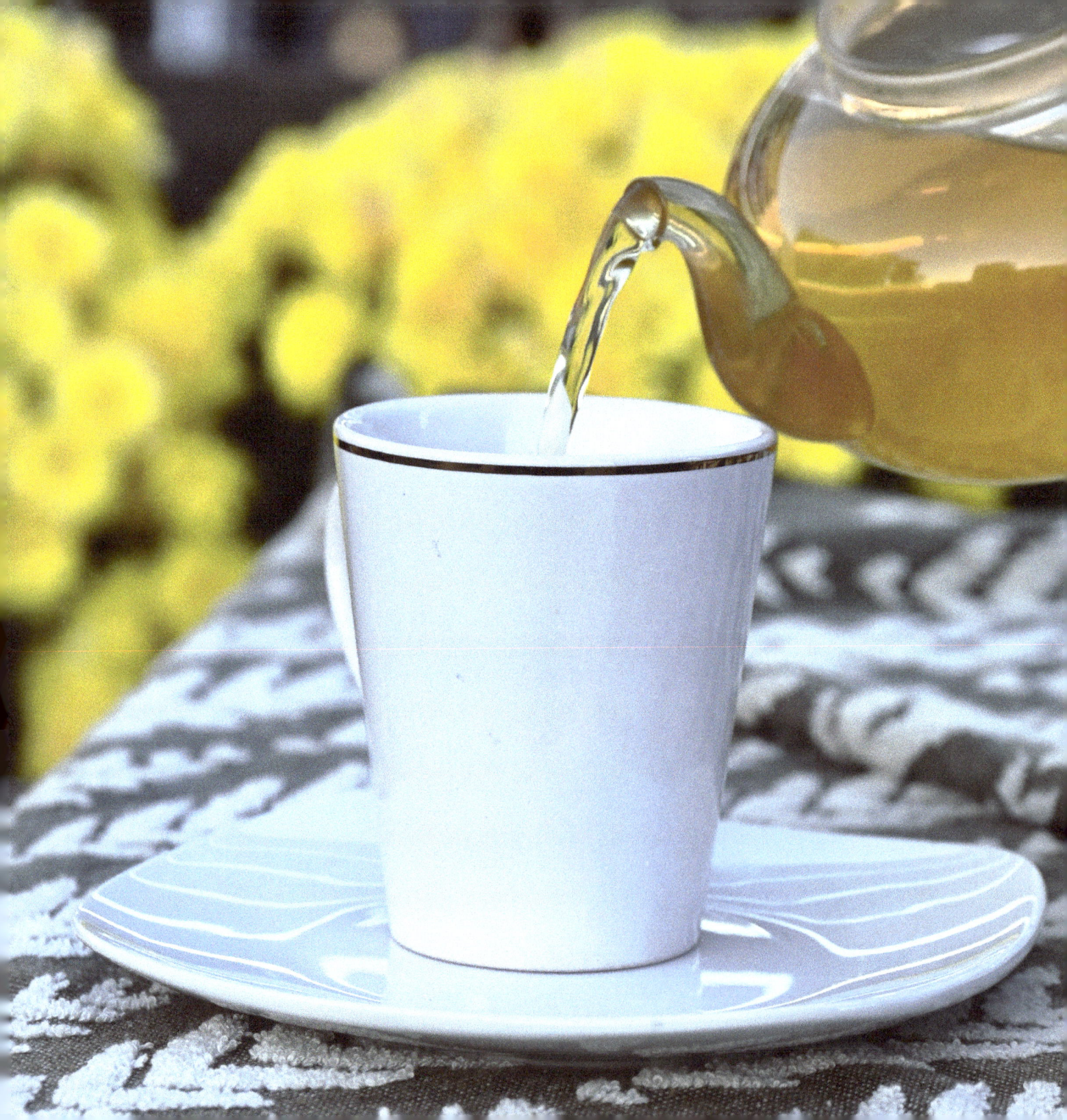

Herbal Teas

Serving size: 1

LIVER PLUS DETOX FORMULA

Plants

- Blessed thistle
- Artichoke
- Dandelion
- Boldo
- Fennel
- Ginger
- Fumitory
- Calendula

Instructions

1. Add 10 g (3.5 oz) each of the first 3
   herbal plants and
   5 g (1.7 oz) each of remaining plants in a jar.
2. Add 500 mL (17 fl oz) of hot water.
3. Let the infusion sit for 15 minutes.

KIDNEY DETOX FORMULA

Plants

Dandelion root

Instructions

1. Add 20 g (0.7 oz) of dandelion root to a jar.
2. Add 200 mL (7 fl oz) of hot water
3. Warm it for 15 minutes and filter before drinking.

COLD FORMULA

Plants

- 10 g (0.35 oz) Blessed Thistle
- 12 g (0.42 oz) Artichoke
- 8 g (0.28 oz) Dandelion
- 5 g (0.17 oz) Boldo
- 5 g (0.17 oz) Fennel
- 7 g (0.25 oz) Ginger
- 6 g (0.21 oz) Fumitory
- 6 g (0.21oz) Calendula

Instructions

1. Mix the leaves in a jar with 200 mL (7 oz) of water.
2. Warm it for 15 minutes and filter before drinking.

STRESS FORMULA 1

Plants

- Oat
- Catnip
- Green anise
- Chamomile
- Melissa
- Indian flowers ➤

STRESS FORMULA 2

Plants

- Chamomile
- Melissa
- Verbena

Instructions

1. Add 10 g (0.35 oz) of each plant to 150 mL (5 fl oz) of water.
2. Warm for 15 minutes and filter before drinking.

IMMUNE SYSTEM BOOST

Plants

Olive leaves

Instructions

1. Add 10 g (0.35 oz) of olive leaves in a jar with 150 mL (5 fl oz) of water.
2. Warm for 15 minutes and filter before drinking.

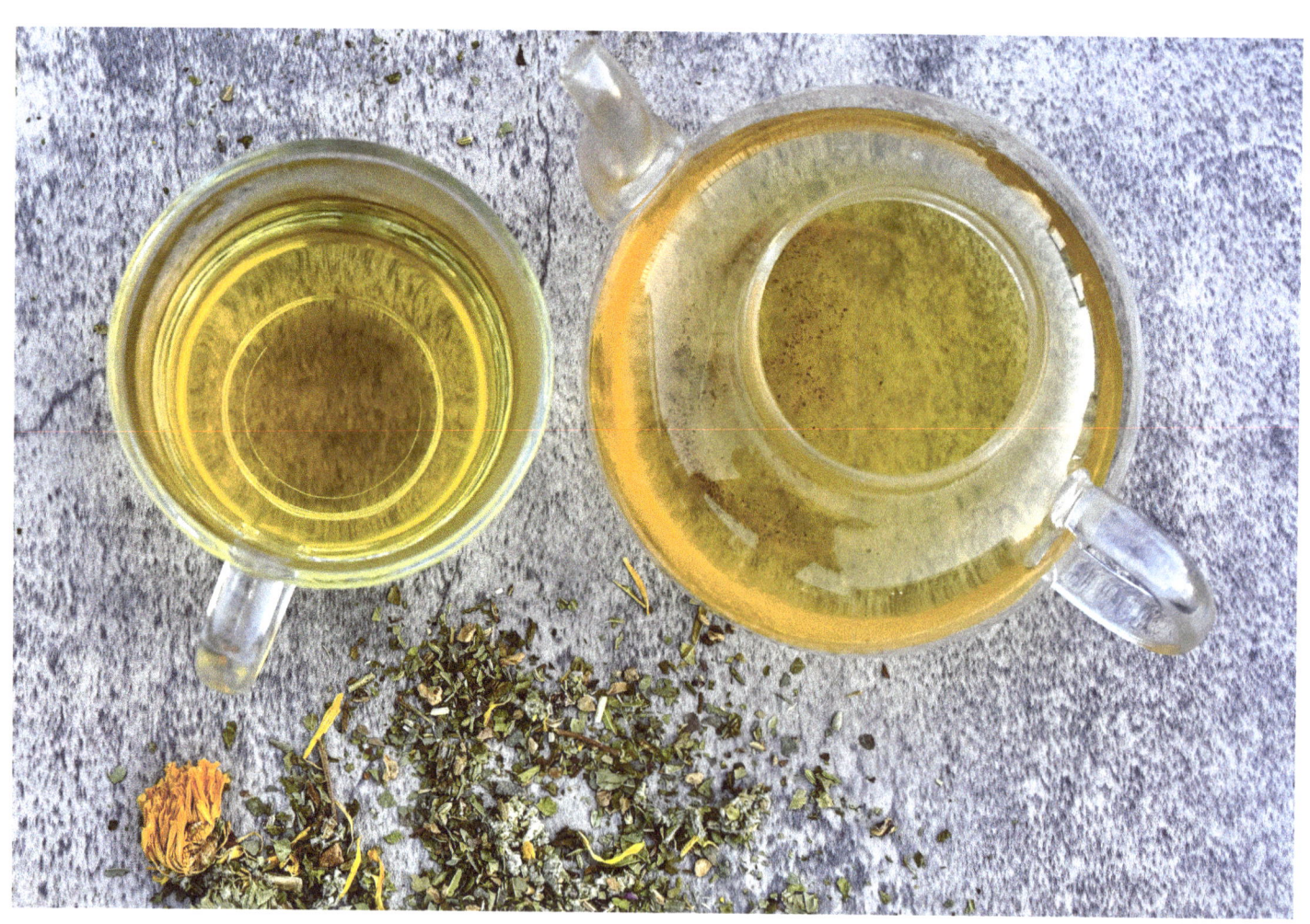

Notes: _____

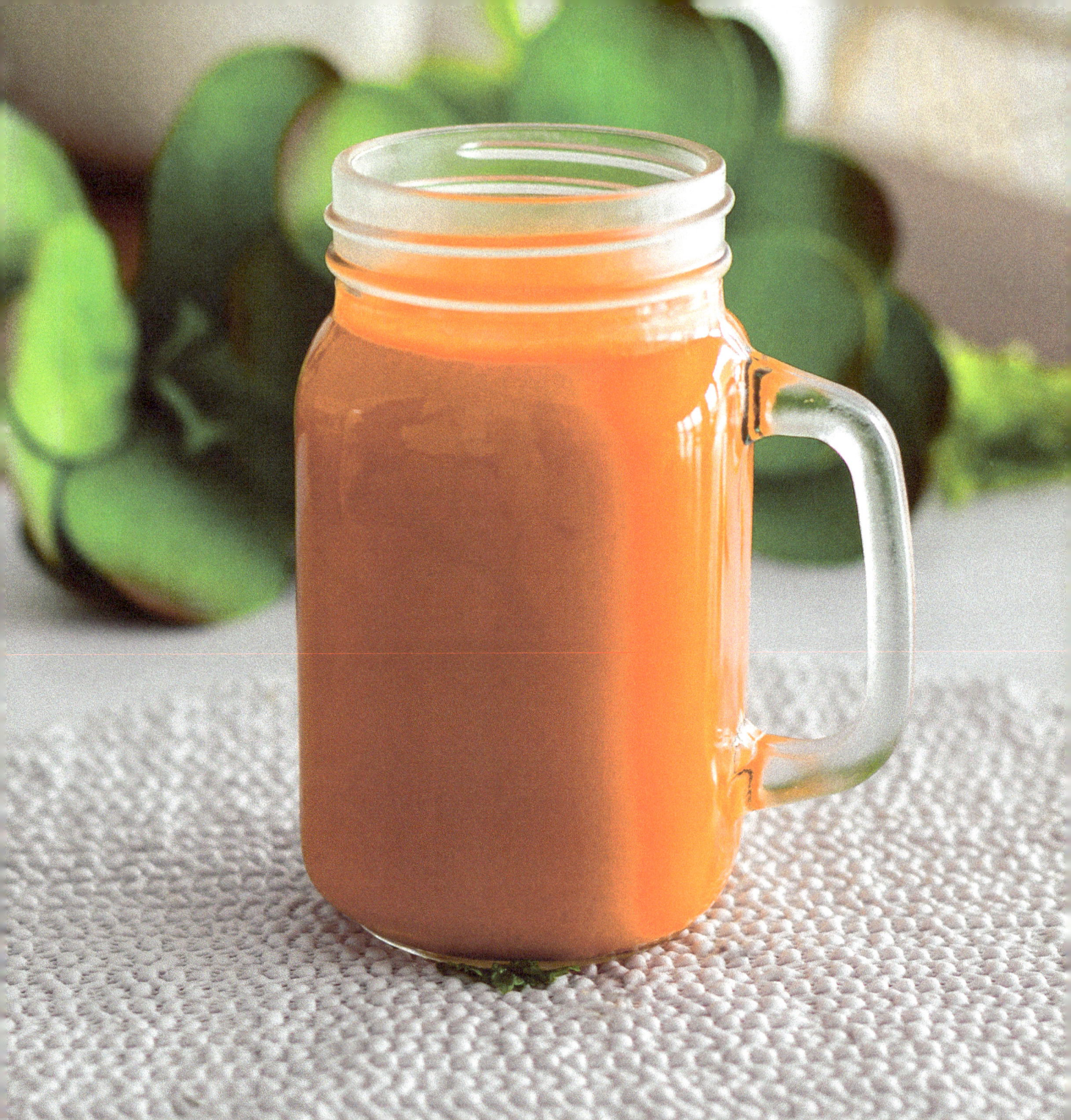

III
RAW NUTRITIOUS JUICES

Raw Living Juices for gut health and energy!

These juices are made fresh and have the wonderful power to alkalinize the body. They will lower the acidity level of the body and reduce inflammation, as long as they are consumed regularly. Nutritious juices should normally be drunk at the beginning of the meal or anytime throughout the day for hydration and to nourish the body with the nutrients it needs.

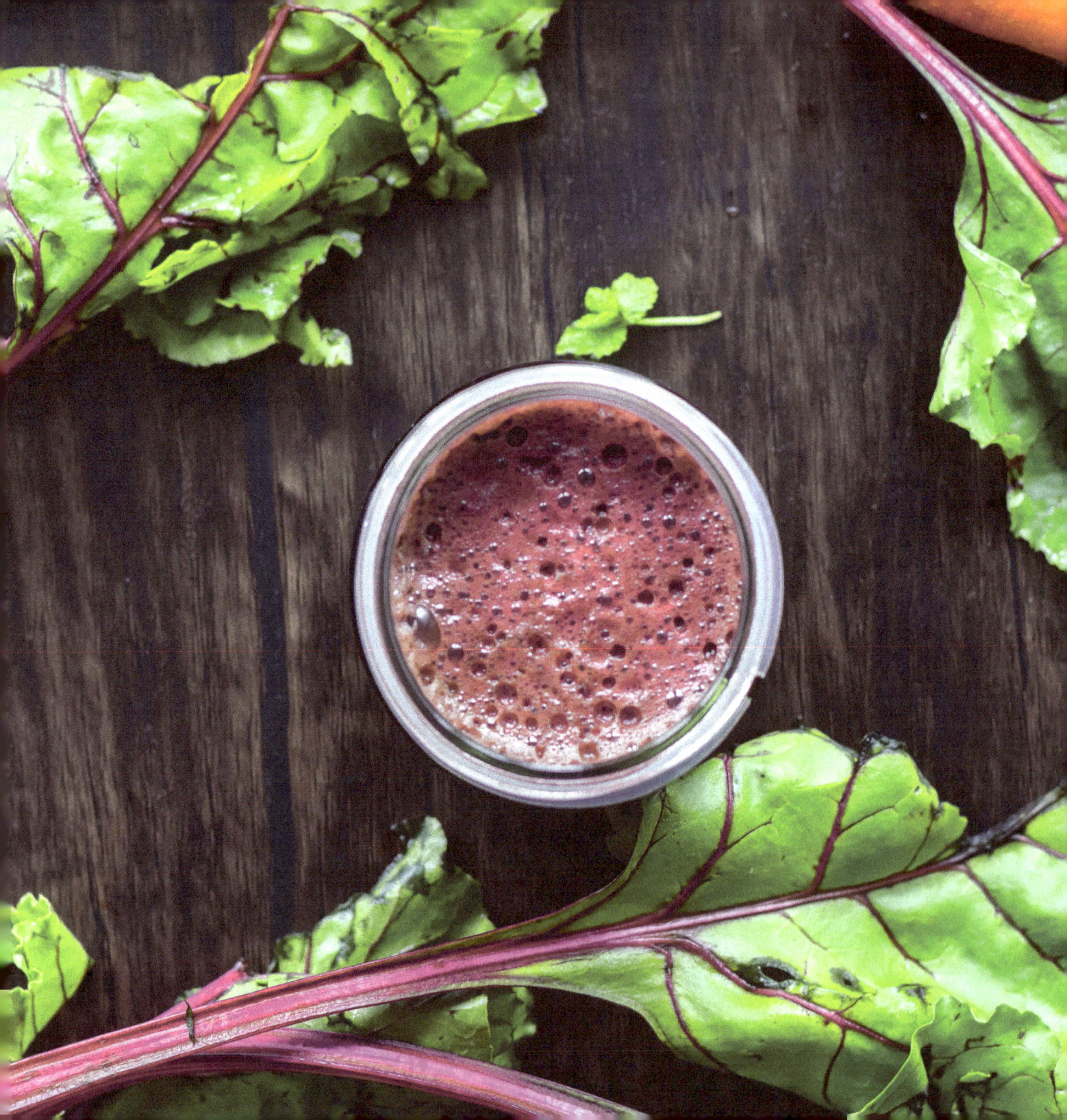

Carrot, Beet & Kale Juice

Serving size: 1

Equipment

- Juice extractor
- Mason jar

Ingredients

- 10 medium carrots
- 4 medium red beets
- 2 bunches kale

Instructions

1. Wash vegetables thoroughly with water or with a combination of water and apple cider vinegar.
2. Place washed vegetables in the juice extractor to get the juice.
3. Add to a mason jar.
4. *Note: If you do not have an extractor, you can use a high-speed blender, but the result will not be quite the same.*
5. Drink the juice fresh immediately to enjoy the benefits of the fresh nutrients.
6. Do not store more than 48 hours in refrigerator.

DID YOU KNOW? *Beets*

Red beetroot is one of the richest vegetables in natural sugar because it contains a high percentage of carbohydrates (sugar), such as sucrose and fructose.

» Excellent antianemic, with an iron content of 1.80 mg/100g.

» High in vitamin C with 30 mg/100g.

» Has alkalizing properties for the blood because of its mineral salts, including potassium, magnesium and calcium.

» Good source of vegetable fiber, which facilitates transit, has a laxative effect and reduces the level of cholesterol in the blood by reducing its absorption in the intestine.

» Beetroot has anticancer properties

» Known for its aperitif effect, increasing the production of gastric juice and toning the stomach.

» Powerful antioxidant that has hepatoprotective effects. In other words, it allows the liver to thrive through self-cleaning.

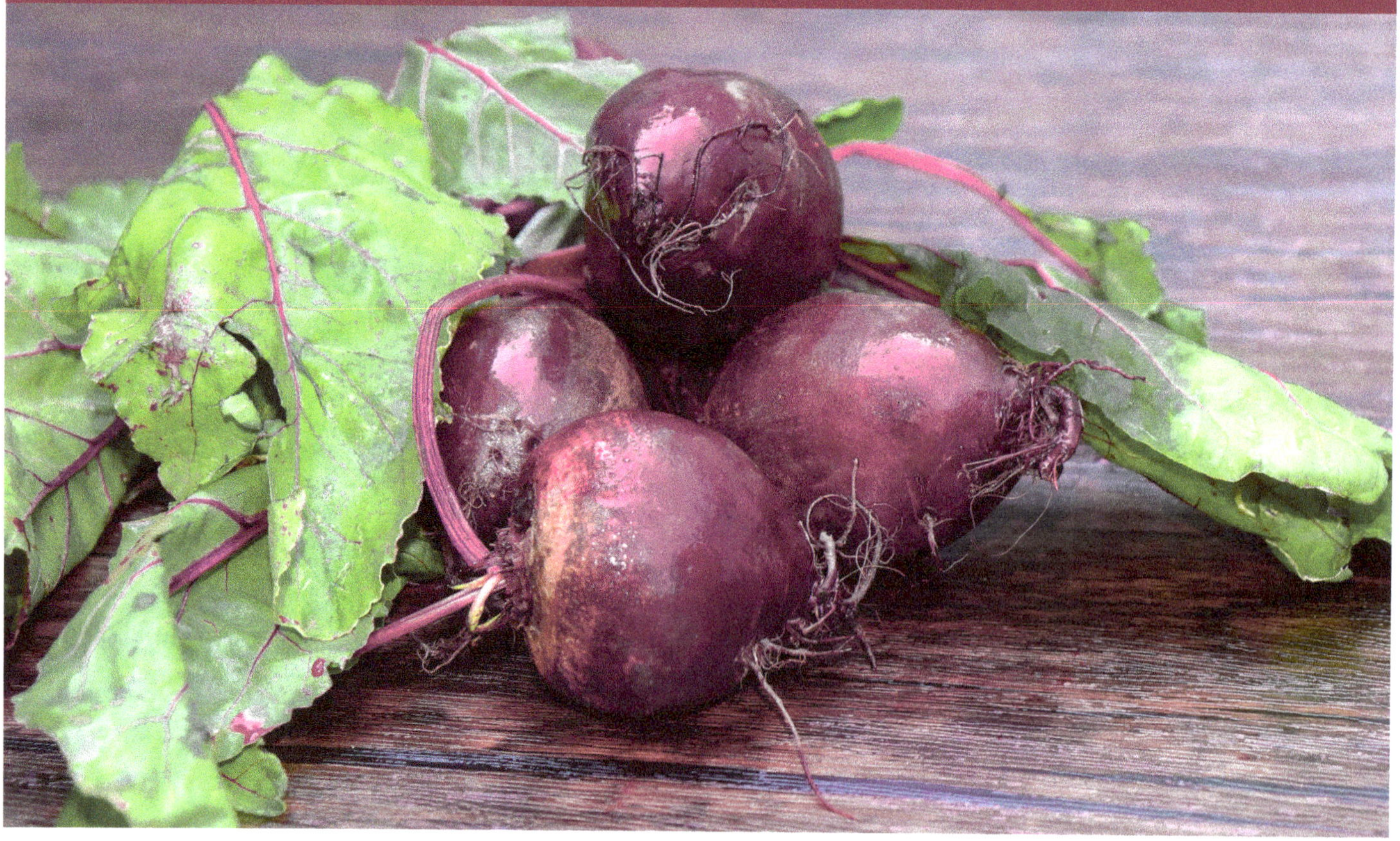

Notes: _____

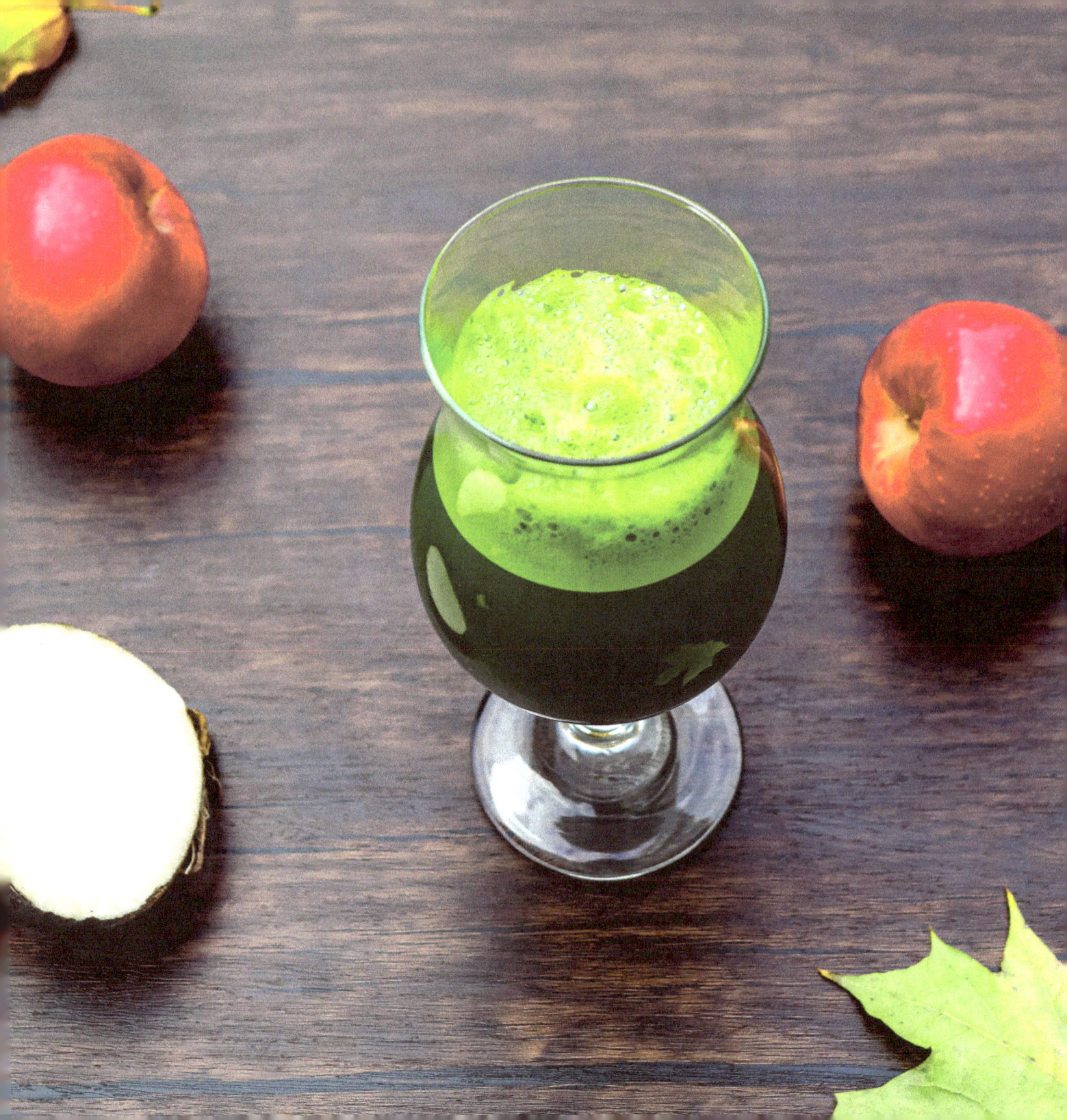

Kale, Apple & Black Radish Juice

Serving size: 1

Equipment

- Mason jar
- Juice extractor

Ingredients

- 2 bundles fresh kale (replace kale with fresh spinach or celery if desired)
- 4 apples
- 1 large black radish

Instructions

1. Wash the vegetables with water and place them in the juice extractor.
2. Extract the juice, add to a mason jar and drink the fresh mixture.
3. To enjoy the benefits of the fresh nutrients, do not store more than 48 hours.

DID YOU KNOW? *Apples*

Apples are the fourth most plentiful fruit in the world after grapes, oranges and bananas.

» Apples are rich in vitamins (C and E) and minerals (potassium and iron).

» Contain an insoluble vegetable fiber called pectin. It is not absorbed by the body. This pectin will act as a "cleaner" to facilitate the elimination of toxins from the stool.

» Known to treat diarrhea and constipation.

» Contains between 1 and 1.5% of organic acids that have an alkalizing effect in the blood and tissues, renewing the intestinal flora and preventing intestinal fermentation.

» Contain flavonoids, which are antioxidants. Flavonoids also prevent the deposition of cholesterol on the walls of the arteries by limiting the arteriosclerosis process (hardening and narrowing of the arteries).

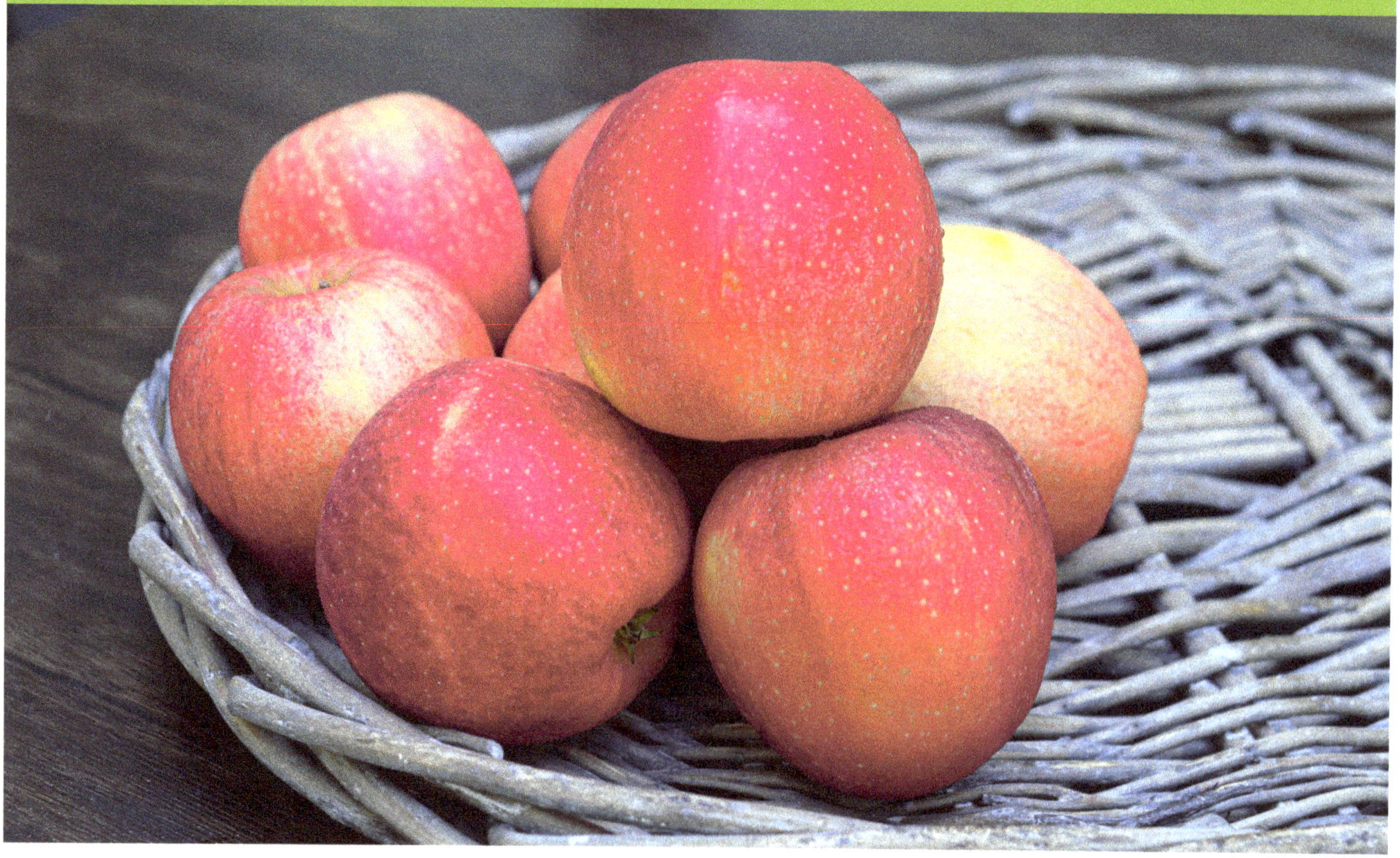

Notes: _____

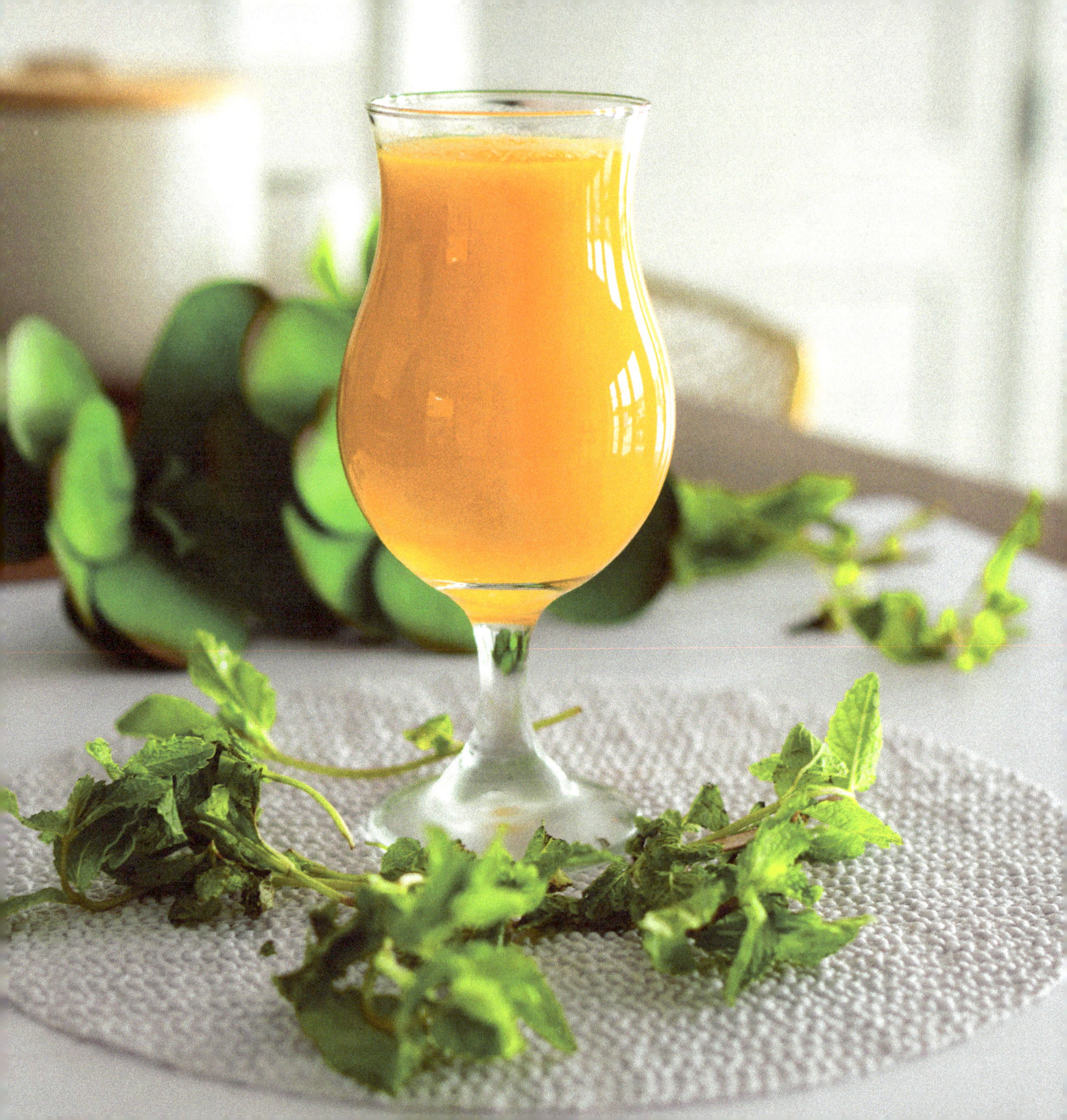

Pineapple, Mango & Kefir Juice

Serving size: 1

STEP 1
FRUIT KEFIR JUICE

Equipment

Mason jar

Ingredients

- 1 qt (1 L) cold water
- 1.7 oz (50 g) organic cane sugar
- 1.7 oz (50 g) fruit kefir
- ½ lime
- 1 piece dried fig

Note: the grains of the fruit kefir (yellowish transparent) are different from those of the milk kefir (white).

Instructions

1. Pour the cold water into a jar. Add the organic cane sugar, fruit kefir, lime and dried fig. Mix well.
2. Cover with a cloth or gauze, held by an elastic band.
3. After 48 hours at room temperature, the drink becomes sparkling. Filter and cool before drinking.

STEP 2

Equipment

- Mason jar
- 1 L glass jar
- Knife
- Juice extractor
- High-speed blender

Ingredients

- 1 large pineapple
- 2 mangoes, ripe and soft
- ½ glass of the juice obtained from the fruit kefir [*see recipe at right*] (*may substitute fruit kefir juice with a probiotic capsule if you prefer*)

Instructions

1. Wash the pineapple with water and peel. Extract the pineapple juice using the juice extractor.
2. Peel the 2 mangoes
3. Add the mango flesh to blender. Blend well.
4. Using high-speed blender, blend the mango mixture, juice of fruit kefir and the pineapple juice extract until smooth.
5. Pour into mason jar. Chill for 15 minutes in refrigerator or drink immediately.

DID YOU KNOW? *Mangoes*

Mangoes are known to nourish the skin and protect the arteries.

- » Contribute to beautiful, healthy skin.

- » Rich in vitamin C, vitamin E, beta carotenes, vitamin B (B1, B2, B6, niacin) and provitamin A.

- » Low in sodium

- » Help with diabetic arterial conditions

- » Recommended in case of eczemas, dermatosis, dry skin and for the prevention of early skin aging.

- » Contain soluble fiber, which is a diuretic.

- » Contains a healthy amount of potassium

- » Recommended to address high blood pressure because of their effects on the arteries and circulation

- » Low glycemic index means mangoes may not dramatically spike blood sugars (though it will raise them over time)

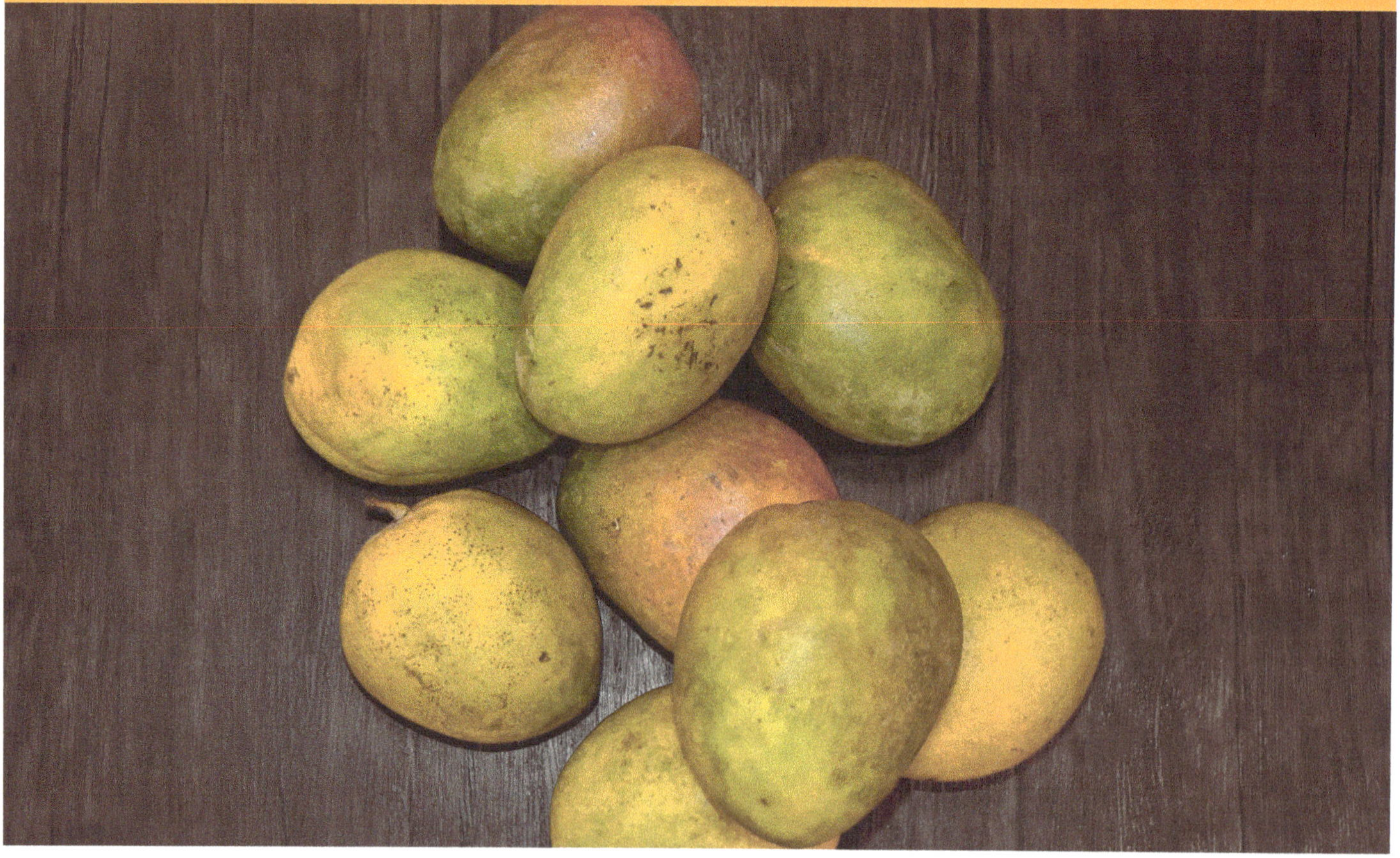

Notes: _____

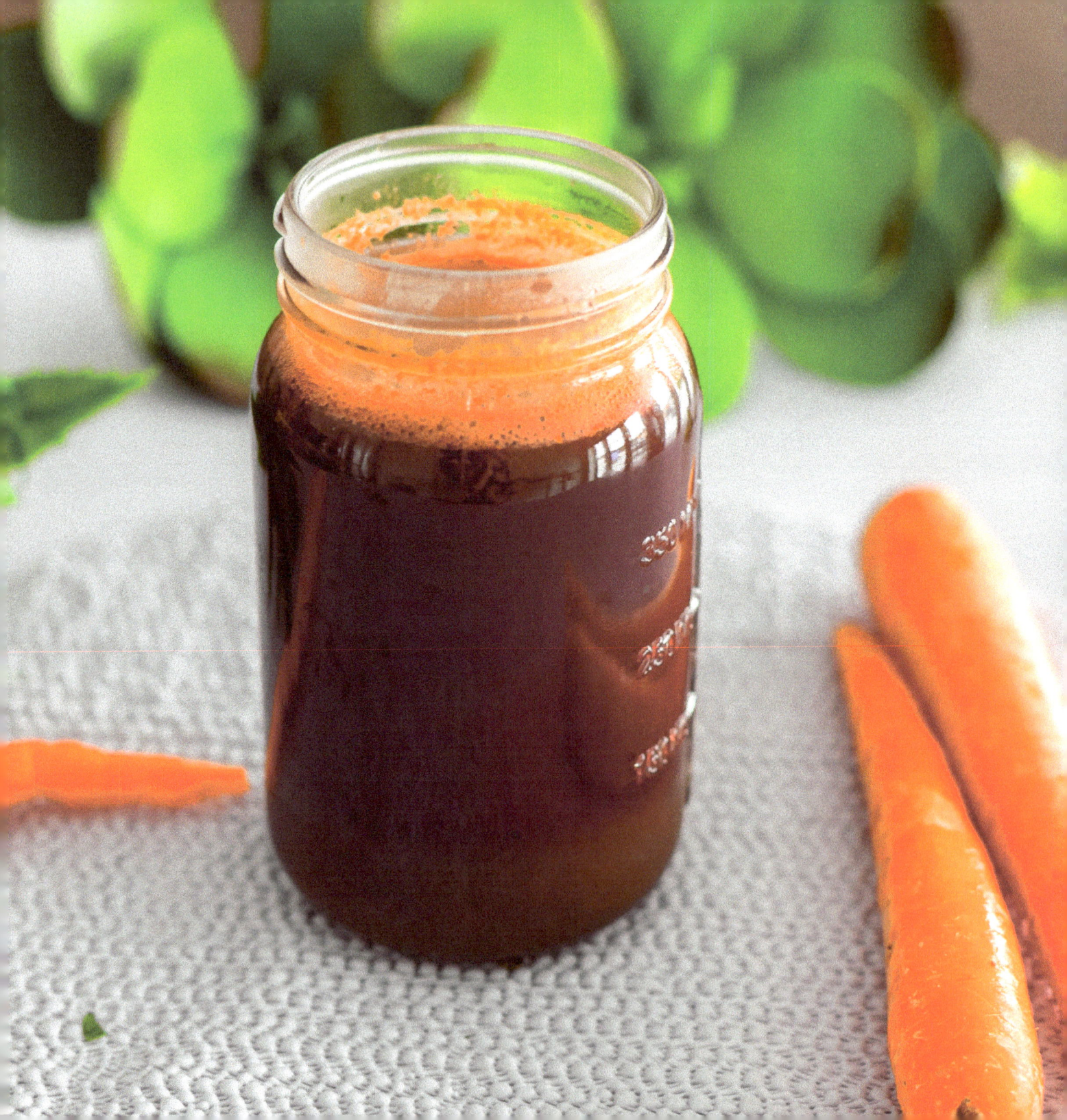

Carrot, Parsley & Black Radish Juice

Serving size: 1

Equipment

- Mason jar
- Knife
- Juice extractor
- High-speed blender

Ingredients

- 5 medium carrots
- ½ raw black radish
- 2 bundles parsley

Instructions

1. Wash carrots, black radish and parsley with water.
2. Place them in juice extractor.
3. Extract the juice.
4. Pour into mason jar.
5. Drink fresh. For those who are not accustomed to black radish, you will notice that it has a particularly strong odor. It is quite normal.

DID YOU KNOW? *Black Radish*

Black radish is the "friend" of the liver par excellence.

» Treats poor bile circulation and digestive disorders by cleansing the gallbladder, liver and intestine

» Reduces inflammation and hypersecretion of the upper respiratory tract (cold, sinusitis, etc.)

» Promotes intestinal transit and blood purification (autolysis of accumulated organic waste and residues that are stagnant in the tissues)

» May help with weight loss

» Contains biological sulfur

» Stimulates nail and hair growth, skin tone and beauty.

» The food supplements of black radish contain antibacterial and antiseptic properties

» Contains isothiocyanates, glucosinolates or raphanin

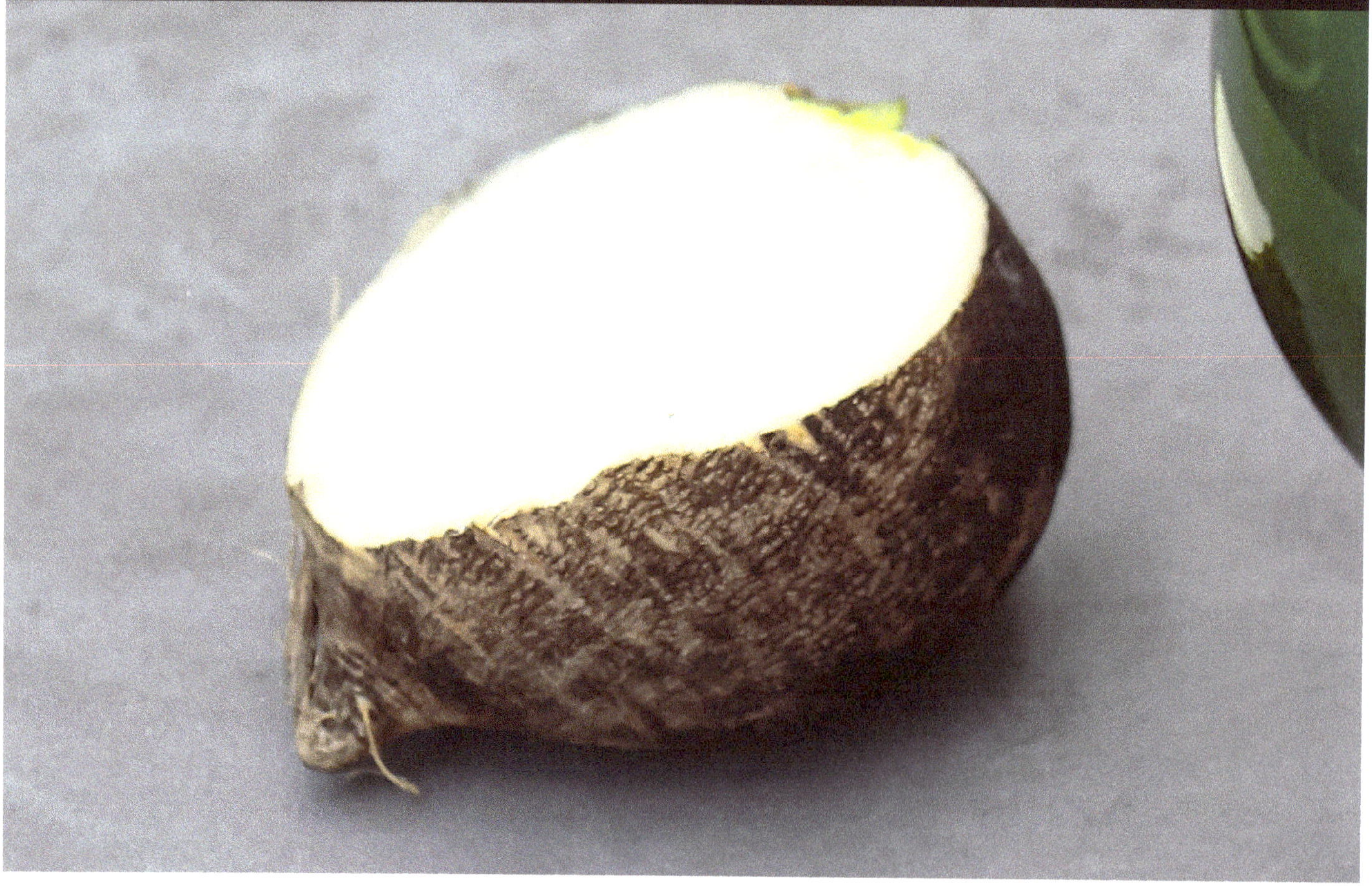

Notes: _____

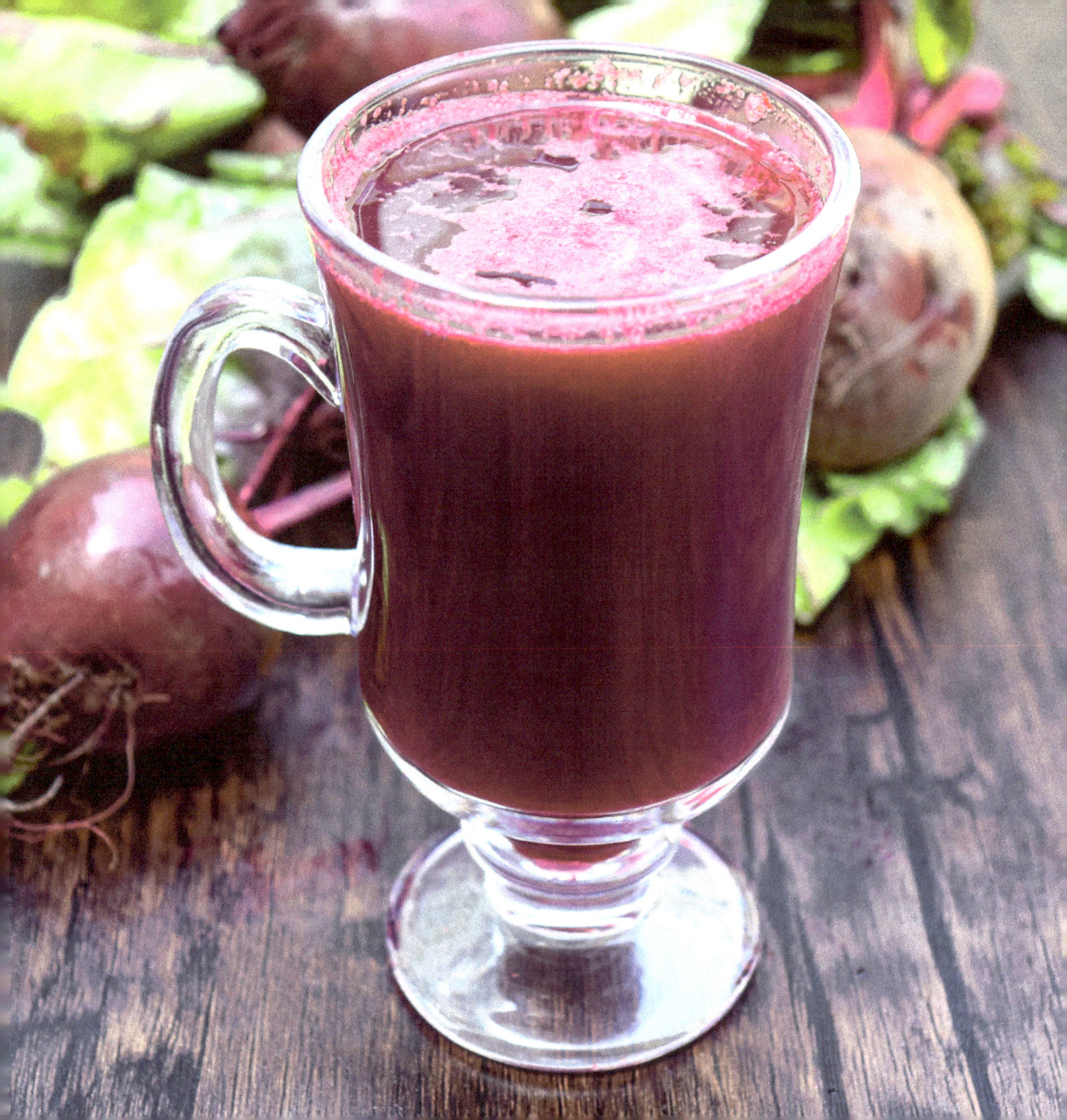

Kale & Beet Juice

Serving size: 1

Equipment
- Mason jar
- Juice extractor

Ingredients
- 1 beetroot
- 2 organic apples
- 1 ginger root
- 1 bunch kale
- 1–2 carrots

Instructions
1. Wash all vegetables thoroughly with water.
2. Add them to a juice extractor.
3. Pour into mason jar. Drink immediately.
4. Store in refrigerator no more than 48 hours.

Based on 95 international studies published recently by the International Journal of Epidemiology, consuming 10 servings of fruits and vegetables per day could prevent nearly 8 million premature deaths worldwide every year. These amounts are generally not consumed by most people around the world.

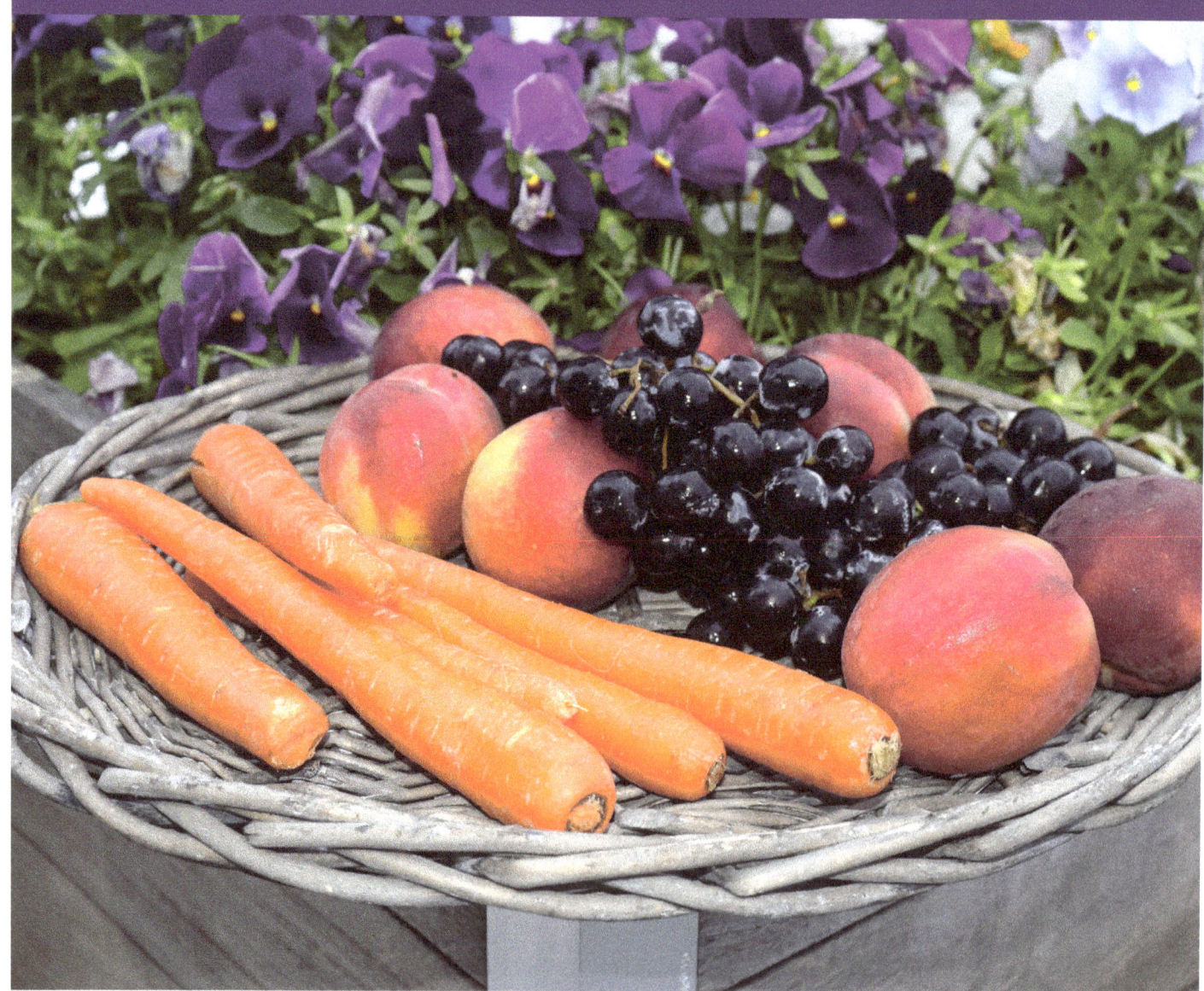

Notes: _____

_____

_____

_____

_____

_____

_____

_____

_____

_____

_____

_____

_____

_____

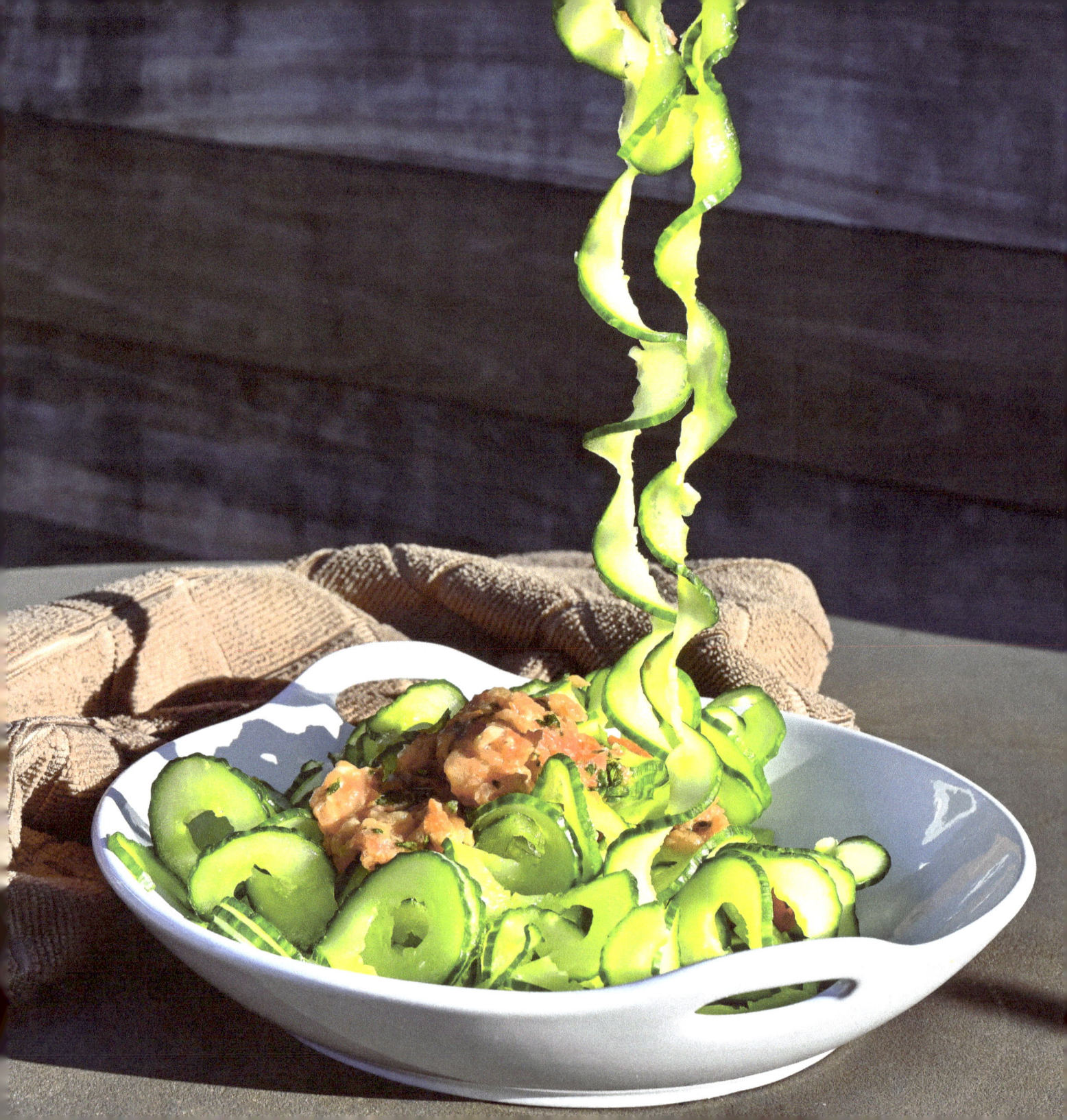

IV
SAVORY RECIPES

The beauty of raw savory food lies in the texture and techniques used to make the food.

Raw living food, like any other type of food, can be made with sweet or savory Ingredients. In this chapter, you will experience various raw food techniques and challenge yourself with simple to advanced recipes.

Raw Living & Fresh Vegetable Salads

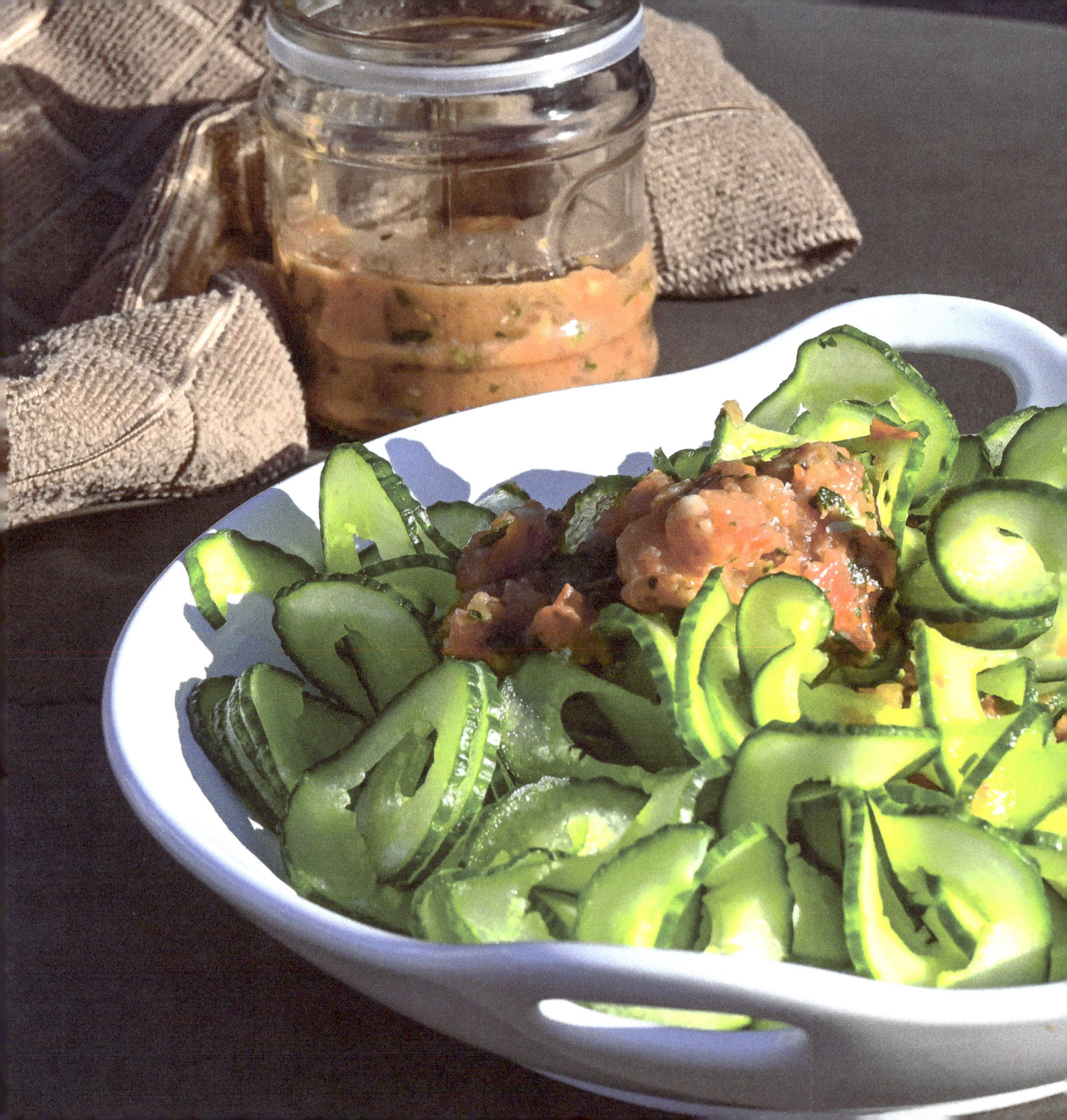

Coodles

Serving size: 1

To enhance your dish, choose one of the seasonings offered in the "Raw Seasonings and Dips" section.

Equipment
- Spiralizer
- Blender
- Glass bowl
- Plate

Ingredients
- 1 Tbsp organic sun-dried tomatoes
- 1 organic tomato, fresh
- 5 basil leaves, fresh
- 5 mint leaves, fresh
- ⅛ cup organic virgin olive oil
- ⅛ cup water, filtered (at room temperature)
- ⅛ tsp Himalayan sea salt
- A pinch of "all spices" (mix of dried spices such as dried parsley, dried basil, mint, coriander, etc. Or make your favorite mix of "all spices!")
  +
- 1 cucumber

Instructions
1. Place first set of ingredients into a high-speed blender and blend until smooth.
2. Add to a glass bowl and set aside.
3. Using the spiralizer, turn the cucumber into noodles. Leave a little bit of the edges of the cucumber to create 2 round shapes of cucumber to be used for the decoration (optional).

ASSEMBLY
1. Place cucumber noodles on a plate. *(Another option is to use a 3.15 inch diameter cake ring mold and place the noodles in the middle to have a nice, round shaped presentation of the noodles.)*
2. Add the round-shaped cucumber to the top (*optional*).
3. Add the tomato sauce in the center of the cucumber noodles.
4. Serve immediately. Can be stored in refrigerator for up to 24 hours.

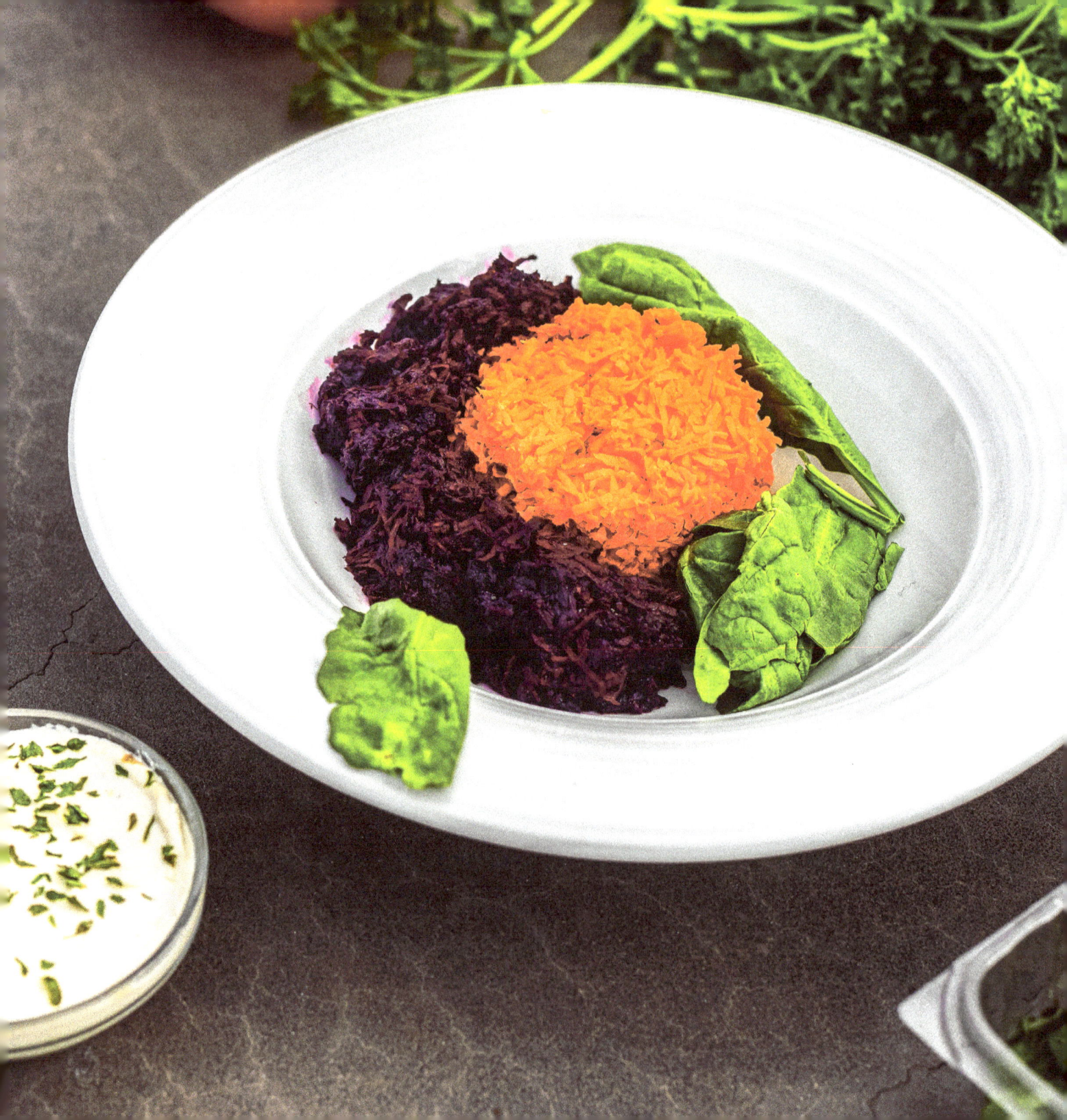

Summer Salad

Serving size: 1

To enhance your dish, you can also opt for a different type of dressing. Check the "Raw Seasonings and Dips" section.

Equipment
- High-speed blender
- Mixing bowl
- Vegetable grater
- Plate
- Sauce dipping bowl

Ingredients for Vegetables
- 3 carrots, fresh
- 1 beetroot
- ½ cup spinach
- 2–4 basil leaves for decoration

Instructions for Vegetables
1. Grate carrots and beets.
2. Toss with the spinach.
3. Add the mixture to a plate.

Ingredients for Dressing
- ½ cup cashews, soaked for 2 hours and rinsed
- 5 Tbsp olive oil
- ¼ tsp salt

Instructions for Dressing
1. Add all dressing ingredients to high-speed blender; blend until smooth. Add a little bit of water as needed.
2. Pour into a sauce dipping bowl.
3. Store in refrigerator for up to 24 hours.

ASSEMBLY
1. Add the dressing in a sauce dipping bowl to the plate containing the grated carrots and beets.
2. Eat immediately or store in refrigerator for up to 3 days.

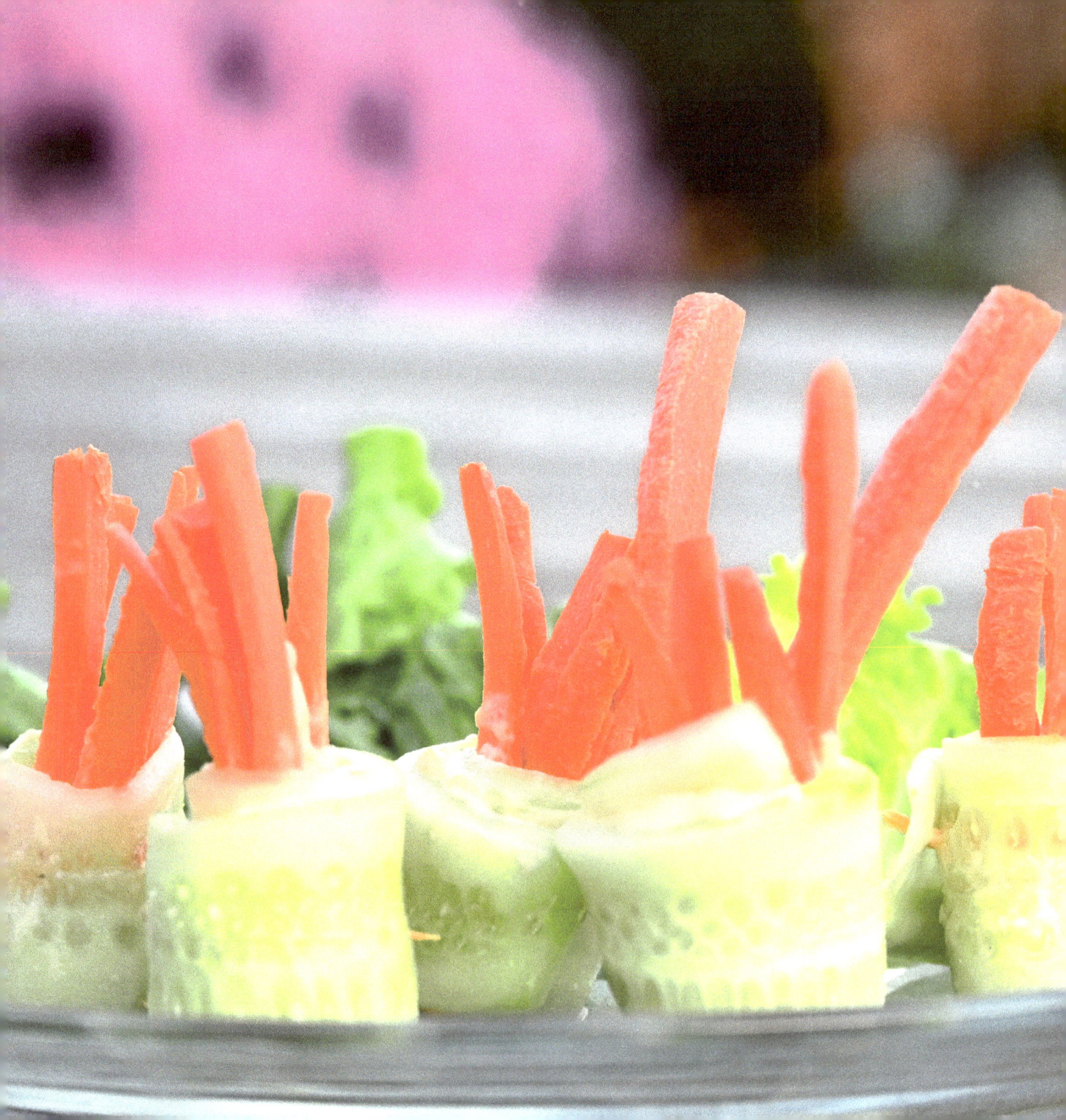

Cucumber Roll

Serving size: 1

Equipment:
- Knife
- Plate
- Spoon
- Toothpick
- Shallow container

Ingredients
- 2 carrots, julienne cut
- 2 cucumbers, fresh
- 1 spinach leaf for decoration

Instructions

1. Using a sharp knife, cut carrots into small sticks as pictured. Add to shallow container and set aside.
2. Cut cucumbers into thin horizontal strips as shown and set aside.
3. Lay down 1 thin layer of a cucumber.
4. Using a spoon, place ½ to 1 Tbsp of a raw cream cheese dressing in the middle *(use the recipe from the "Raw Seasonings and Dips" section).*
5. Add julienne carrots on top of cream cheese sauce.
6. Roll slowly and secure with toothpick.
7. Repeat steps 1–5 until all the cucumber strips are used.

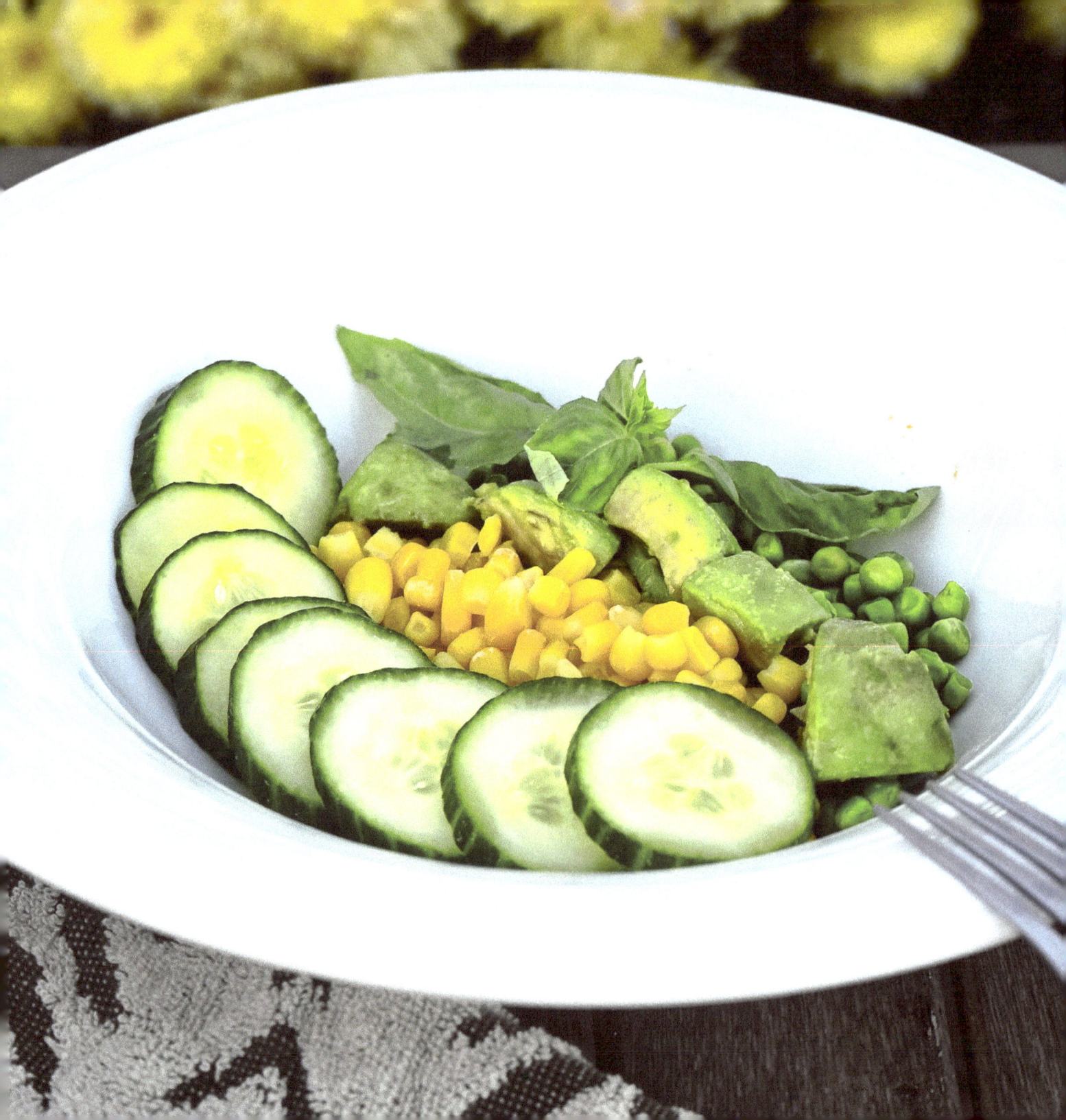

Cucumber & Avocado Salad

Serving size: 1

Equipment
- Knife
- Mixing bowl
- Spatula
- Plate

Ingredients
- 1 cucumber
  +
- 1 avocado (not too ripe)
  +
- ½ onion
- ½ cup of sweet corn
- ¼ cup sweet peas
  +
- 1 Tbsp walnut oil
- 1 Tbsp carrot oil
- 1 Tbsp hemp oil
- ¼ tsp Himalayan sea salt

Instructions
1. Cut cucumber into round slices.
2. Remove skin from avocado and cut into cubes. Set aside.
3. Dice onion.
4. Add onions, sweet corn and peas to mixing bowl.
5. Add oils and salt. Mix well using spatula.
6. Add cucumber and avocado to a plate.
7. Pour the mix of oils on it. Serve immediately.
8. *Optional*: Dried nettle leaves may be added.

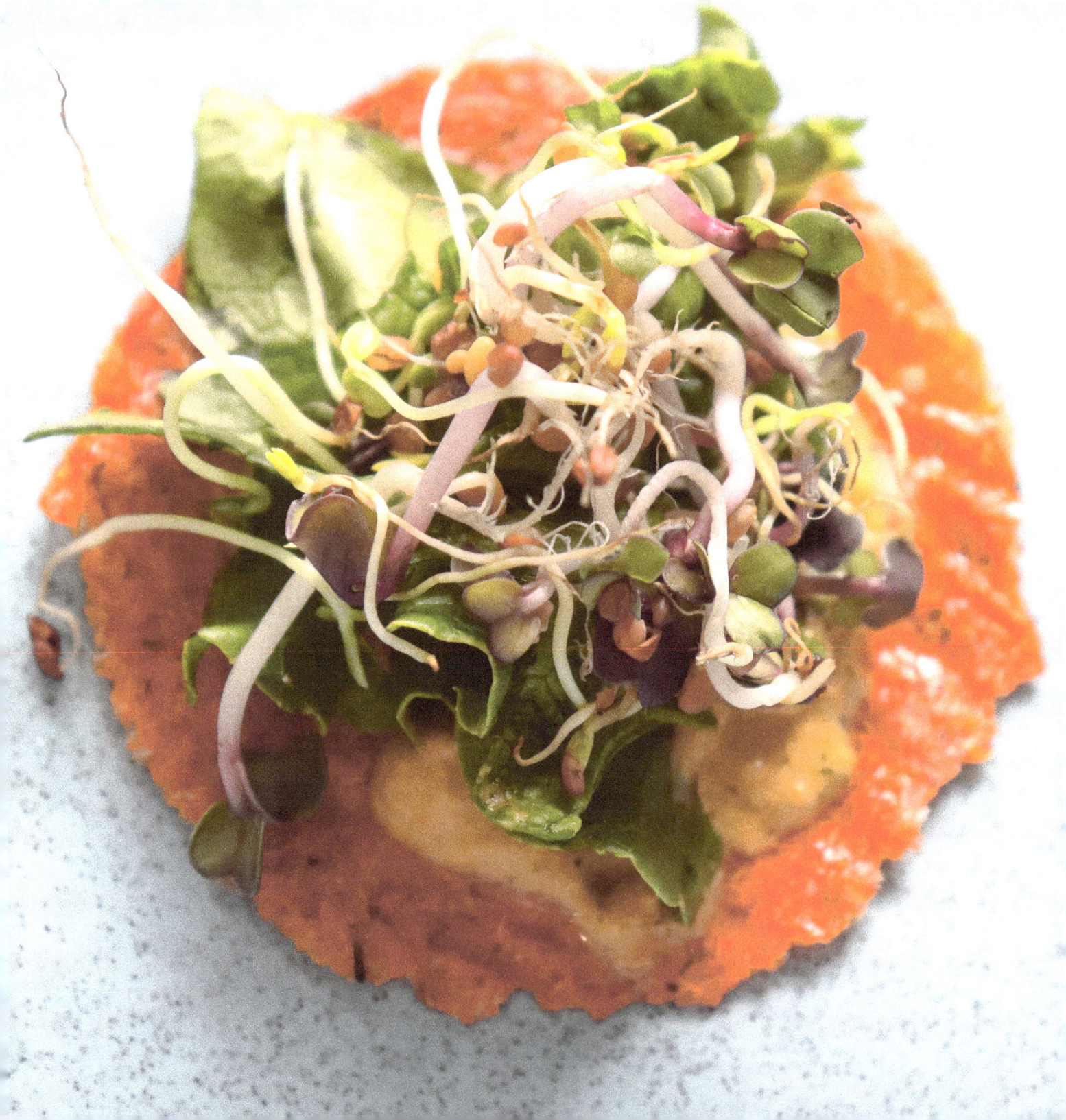

Raw Tacos Recipe

Serving size: 1

This recipe will be made in 5 steps:

STEP 1: SPROUTS

STEP 2: TOMATO SAUCE

STEP 3: RAW CHEESE

STEP 4: CRUST

STEP 5: ASSEMBLY

STEP 1: MAKING THE SPROUTS

Equipment

- Mason jar
- Sprouting jar with lid
- Strainer
- Mixing bowl

Ingredients

- 2 Tbsp sprouted seeds of salad mix (mix of radish, kale and broccoli) or any mix of your choice
- Filtered water (enough to submerge seeds)

Instructions

1. Add sprouted seeds to a mason jar and pour filtered water into it. Let it sit on the counter for 4 to 5 hours. The seeds must be submerged in the water. *As a rule of thumb, the quantity of water must be at least twice that of seeds.*

2. After 4 to 5 hours, using a strainer, rinse the seeds with water and pour the soaked seeds into a sprouting jar with a lid.

3. Make sure the sprouting jar is well closed and turn it upside down to let the remaining water out. *Be sure to have the sprouting jar propped against a wall at a 45° angle because the seeds will not survive the sprouting process if they retain too much moisture.*

4. Rinse the seeds 2 to 3 times a day for 4 to 5 days, returning them to the same position in the jar after each rinse. *Note: The jar MUST never be left horizontally throughout the sprouting process to avoid excessive moisture in the seeds.*

5. When your seeds start sprouting, they will become yellow then green, and your jar will tend to be full.

6. When you get to that stage, put the jar in the refrigerator. ➤

STEP 2: THE TOMATO SAUCE

Equipment
- Blender
- Mixing bowl

Ingredients
- 1 fresh tomato, organic
- 2 dried tomatoes
- ⅛ cup filtered water
- ½ tsp thyme seasoning
- ½ tsp fresh parsley
- ⅛ tsp Himalayan sea salt

Instructions
1. Blend all sauce ingredients in a high-speed blender until smooth.
2. Pour into a mixing bowl.
3. Dehydrate at 115°F (46°C) for at least 2 hours and set aside.
4. You can store tomato sauce in the refrigerator for up to 1 week.

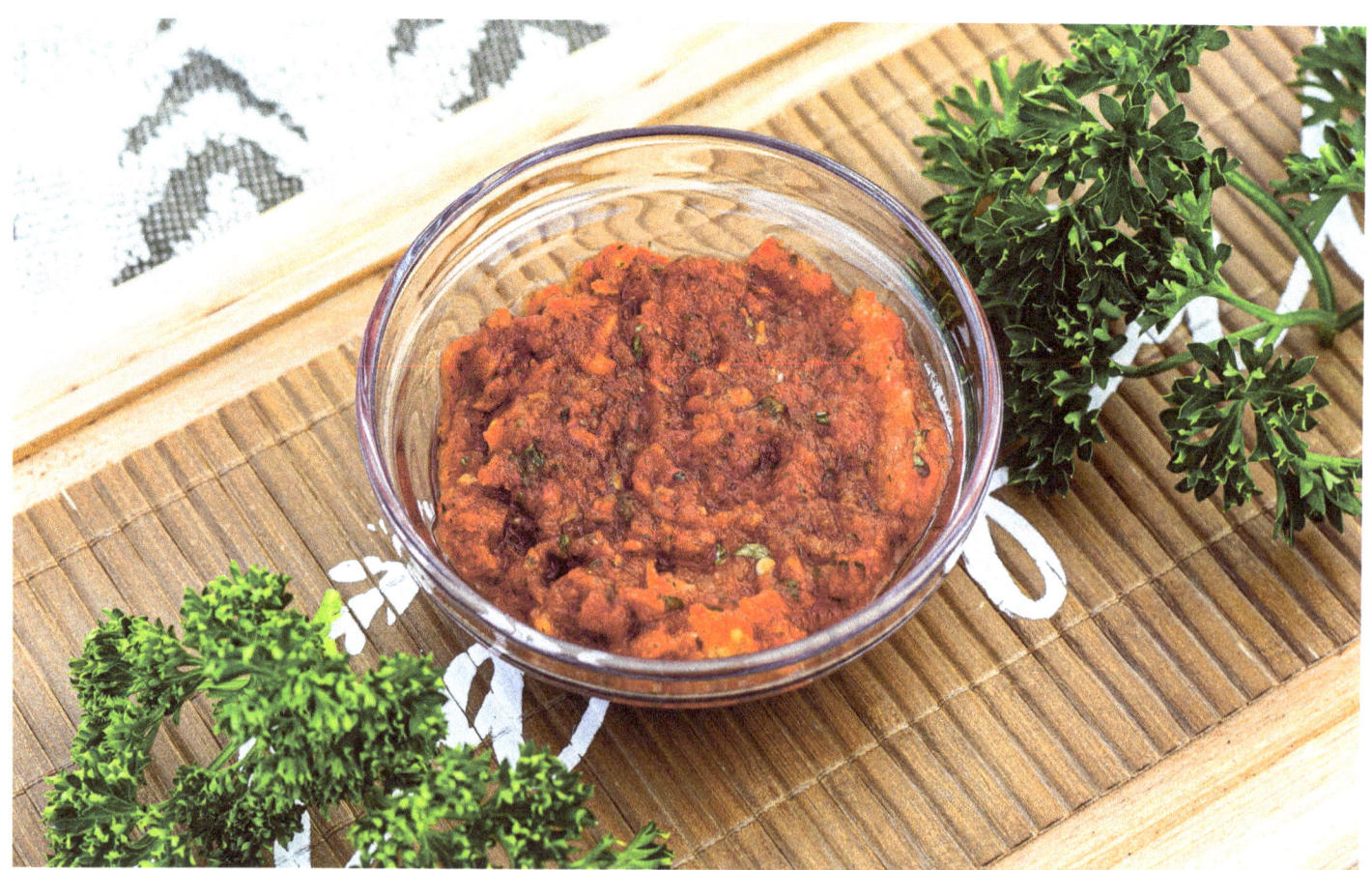

STEP 3: RAW CHEESE

Equipment

- Blender
- Mixing bowl
- Parchment paper
- Cutting board
- 3 inch ring mold
- Ring mold pushers

Ingredients

- ½ cup raw cashews, soaked for 8 hours and rinsed
- ½ Tbsp orange juice
- ½ Tbsp cold pressed olive oil
- ⅛ tsp Himalayan sea salt
- 7 Tbsp water, filtered
  +
- ½ cup dried parsley flakes for decoration

Instructions

1. Soak cashew nuts for 8 hours or overnight. Rinse well.
2. Add cashews to blender along with all ingredients of the raw cheese. Blend until smooth.
3. Line a cutting board with parchment paper and place the ring molds on top.
4. Pour the mixture into the ring molds.
5. Tap the cutting board (with the ring mold and cheese) gently onto the counter to remove air bubbles.
6. Dehydrate for 8 hours at 115°F (46°C) at least or overnight.
7. Then refrigerate for 1 hour.
8. Remove from the refrigerator.
9. Using the ring mold pushers, remove cheese from ring mold.
10. Pour dried parsley flakes into a bowl.
11. Roll cheese in parsley flakes covering both sides.
12. You can keep this in freezer for up to 2 weeks. ➤

STEP 4: CRUST

Equipment
- Knife
- Blender
- Mixing bowl
- Spatula
- Spoon
- 4 ring molds
- Dehydrator
- Parchment paper

Ingredients
- 1 large carrot, raw
- ½ cup filtered water
- ½ tsp dried thyme
- ⅛ tsp Himalayan sea salt
- 1 tsp cold pressed olive oil
- 1 tsp dried parsley
  +
- ⅛ cup psyllium husk

Instructions
1. Using a knife, dice carrots to facilitate blending process.
2. Add all crust ingredients to blender *(except the psyllium husk)*.
3. Blend until smooth.
4. Place mixture in mixing bowl.
5. Incorporate psyllium husk to the mixing bowl; mix well using a spatula.
6. Line a dehydrator sheet with parchment paper and place ring molds on top.
7. Using a spoon, pour equal amounts of mixture into 4 ring molds (about 1 tsp to have thin crusts).
8. If you have some mixture left, repeat the same process with another set of ring molds. The mixture should now stick to the parchment paper.
9. Gently remove the ring molds.
10. Dehydrate at 115°F (46°C) for 4 hours.
11. After 4 hours of dehydration, flip the crusts.
12. Dehydrate for an additional 4 hours.
13. Check periodically to make sure crust is supple, pliable and not too dry. Remove when crust is supple.

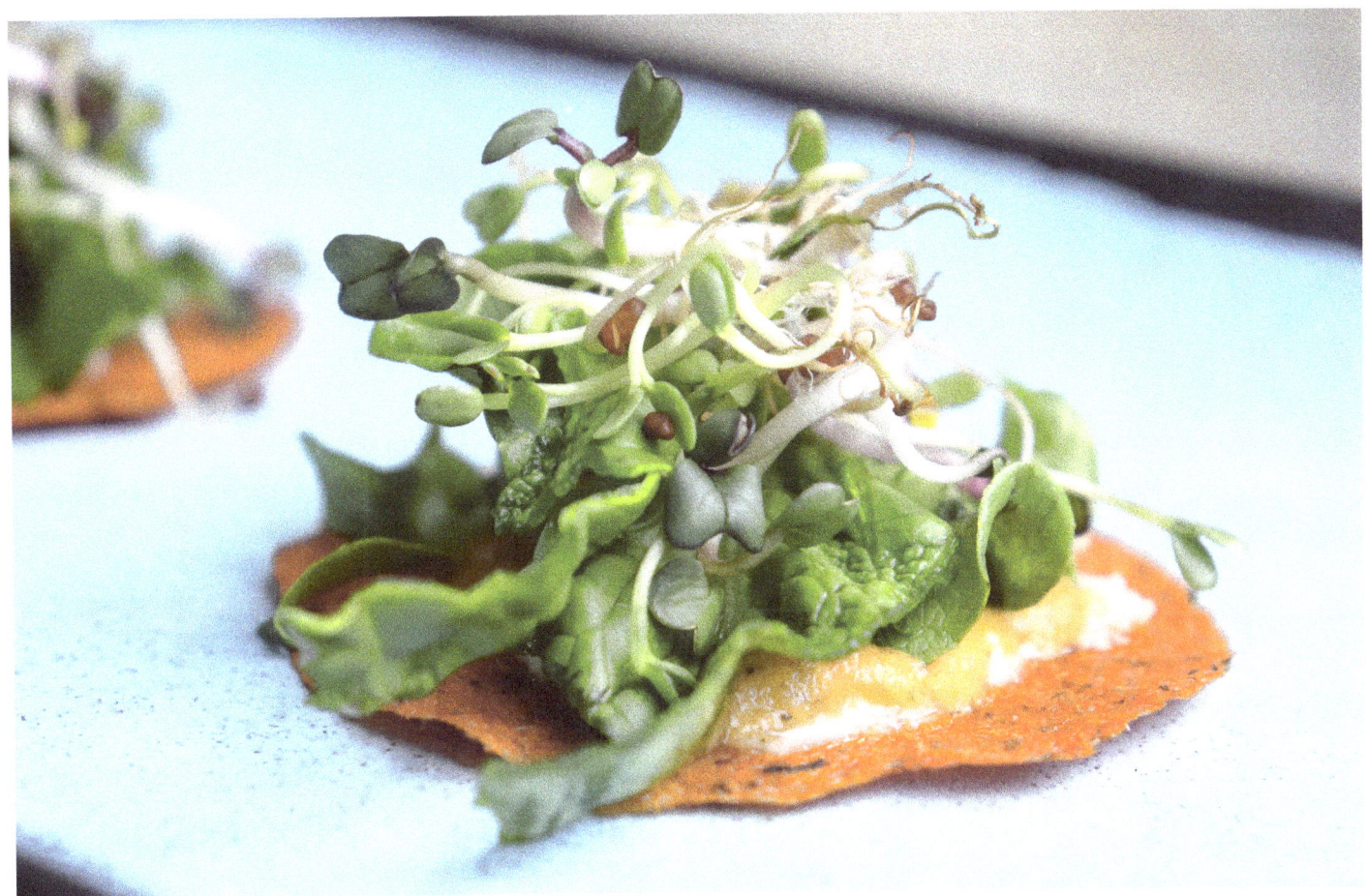

STEP 5: ASSEMBLY

Ingredients

- 4 dehydrated crusts
- 4 Tbsp tomato sauce
- 4 Tbsp raw cheese
- 4 leaves lettuce, chopped
- 4 Tbsp salad mix sprouts (*from Step 1*)

Instructions

1. Line the 4 crusts on the table.
2. Pour 1 tablespoon of tomato sauce on each crust.
3. Cut cheese into pieces and add about 1 tablespoon on top of the tomato sauce for each taco.
4. Add about 1 tablespoon of fresh lettuce.
5. Top with a bit of sprout and enjoy.
6. Store assembled tacos in refrigerator for up to 24 hours.

DID YOU KNOW? *Sprouts*

Micro-sprouts fall into the category of vegetables, and it is still early to accurately determine the exact minimum amount to consume daily but it is known that they are highly rich in nutrients and enzymes compared to their mature version. For example, kale sprouts have been shown to contain 100 times more enzymes and nutrients than the mature kale. Similarly, red cabbage sprouts contain 69 times more vitamin K, 40 times more vitamin E and 6 times more vitamin C than the mature red cabbage. Thus, the consumption of micro-sprouts can make a significant difference in helping to fill nutritional deficiencies.

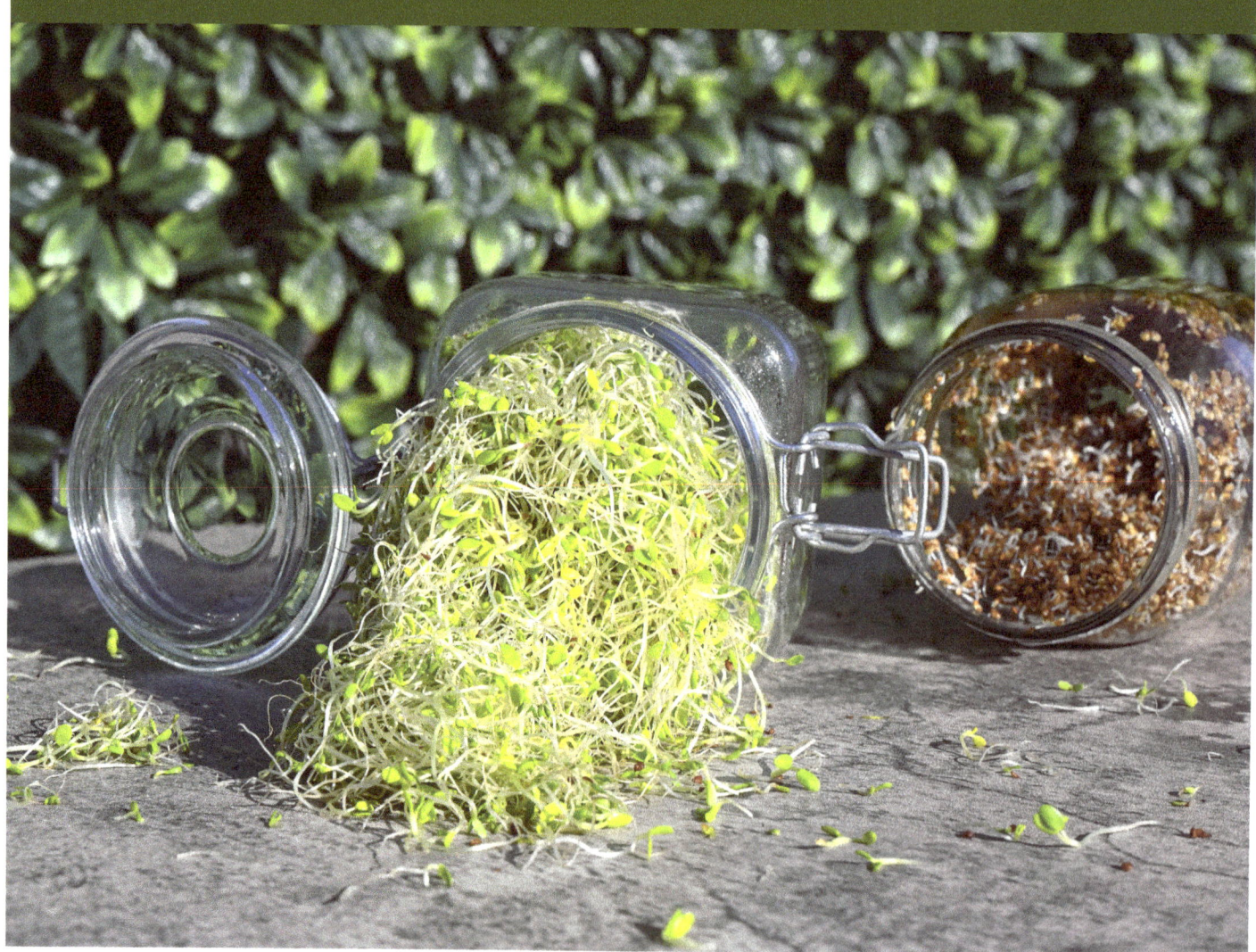

Notes: _____

_____

_____

_____

_____

_____

_____

_____

_____

_____

_____

_____

_____

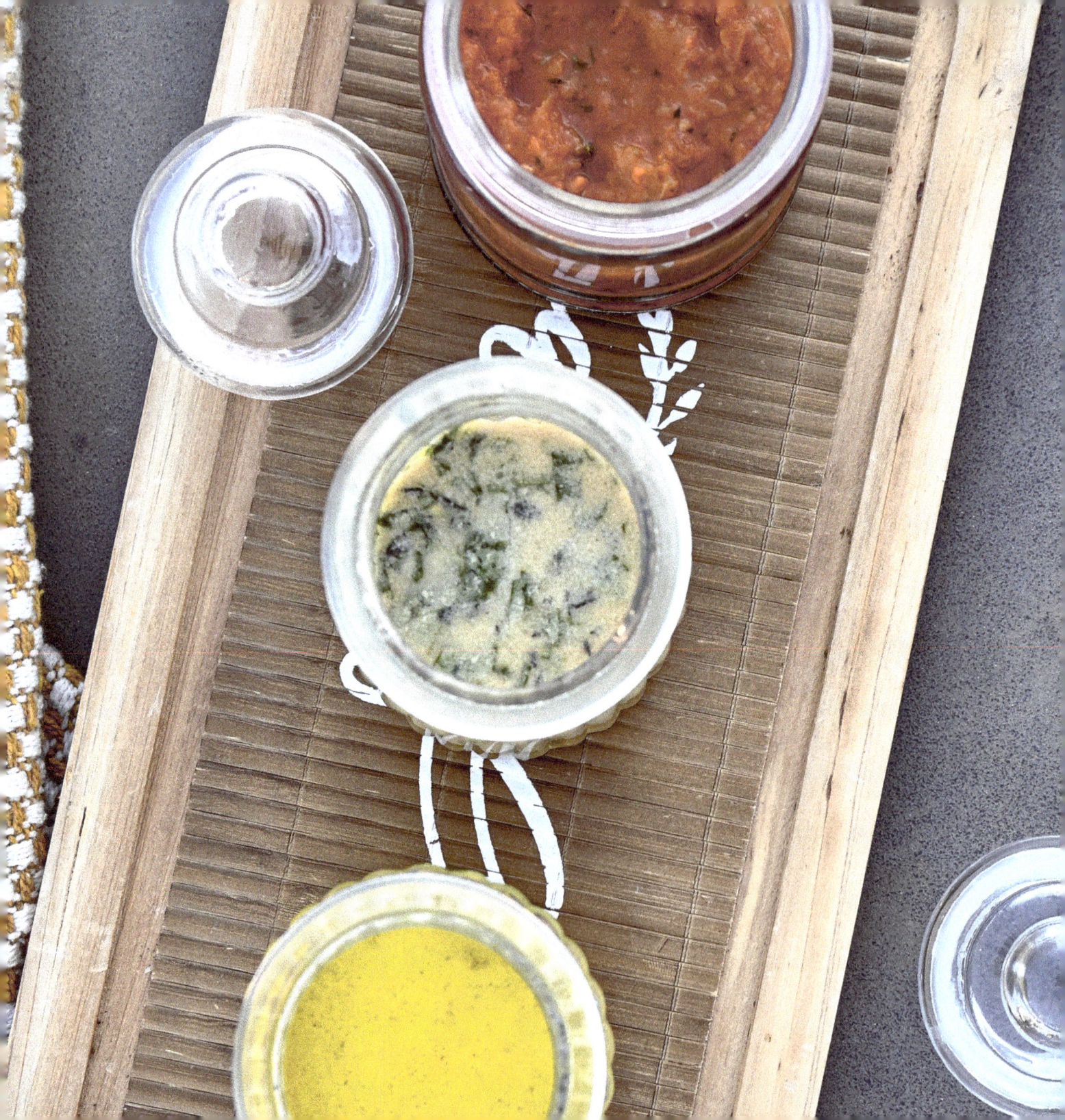

V
DIPS & SEASONING

Nothing beats a nice seasoning to accompany and embellish our dishes!

Sauces upgrade the taste of recipes and are a great opportunity to include herbs and spices on our plate. Note that the same sauce can go with different savory raw recipes.

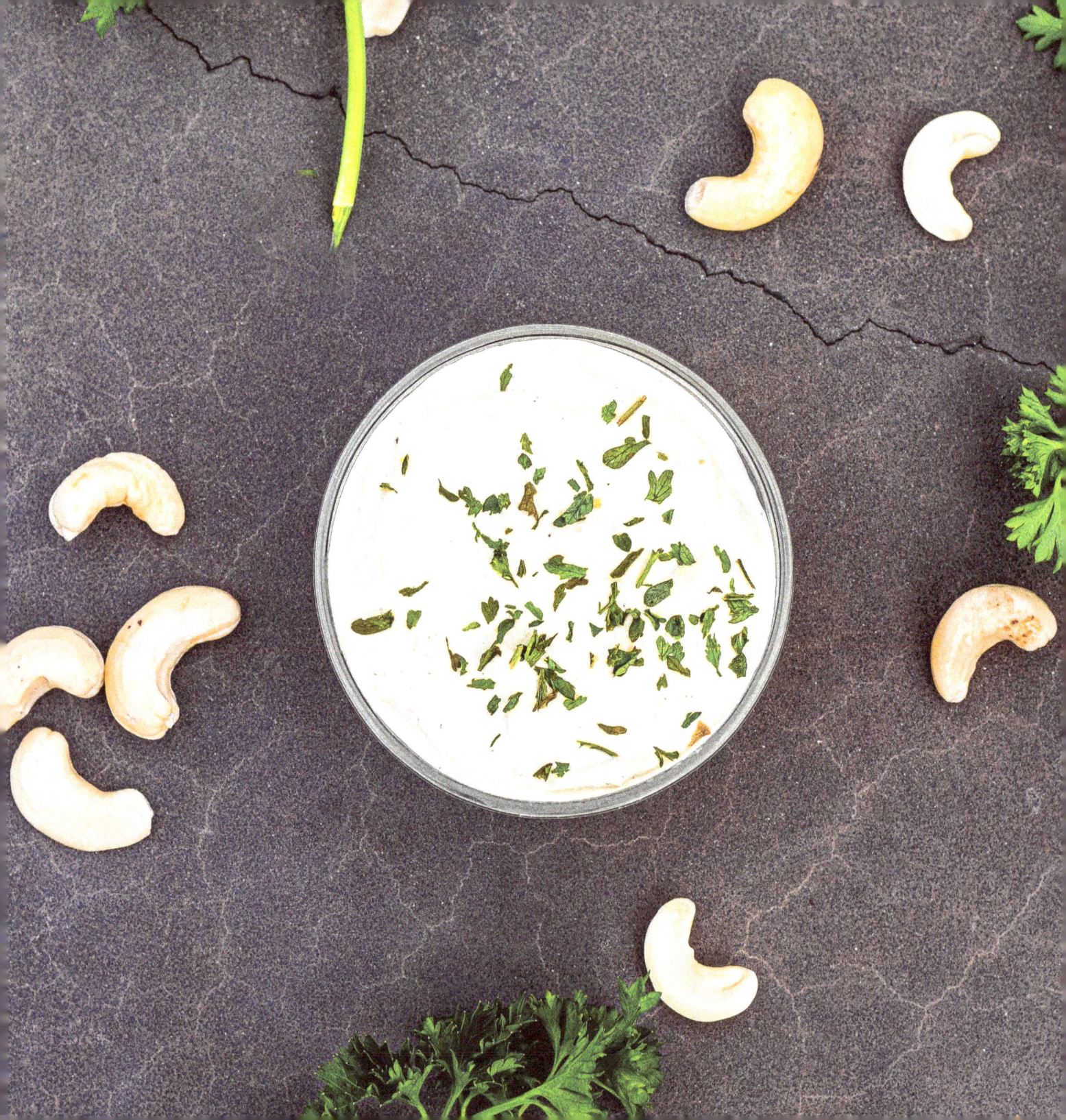

Raw Dipping Cream Cheese Sauce

Serving size: 8

Equipment

- Shallow container
- High-speed blender

Ingredients

- 2 cups raw cashews, soaked for 2 hours and rinsed
- ¾ cup water, room temperature
- 2 Tbsp olive oil
- 1 Tbsp tahini
- 1 tsp Dijon mustard
- ½ tsp ground black pepper
- ¼ tsp Himalayan sea salt

Instructions

1. Add all ingredients to high-speed blender.
2. Blend until smooth.
3. Pour into a shallow container.
4. Serve immediately. Can be stored for 1 week in refrigerator.

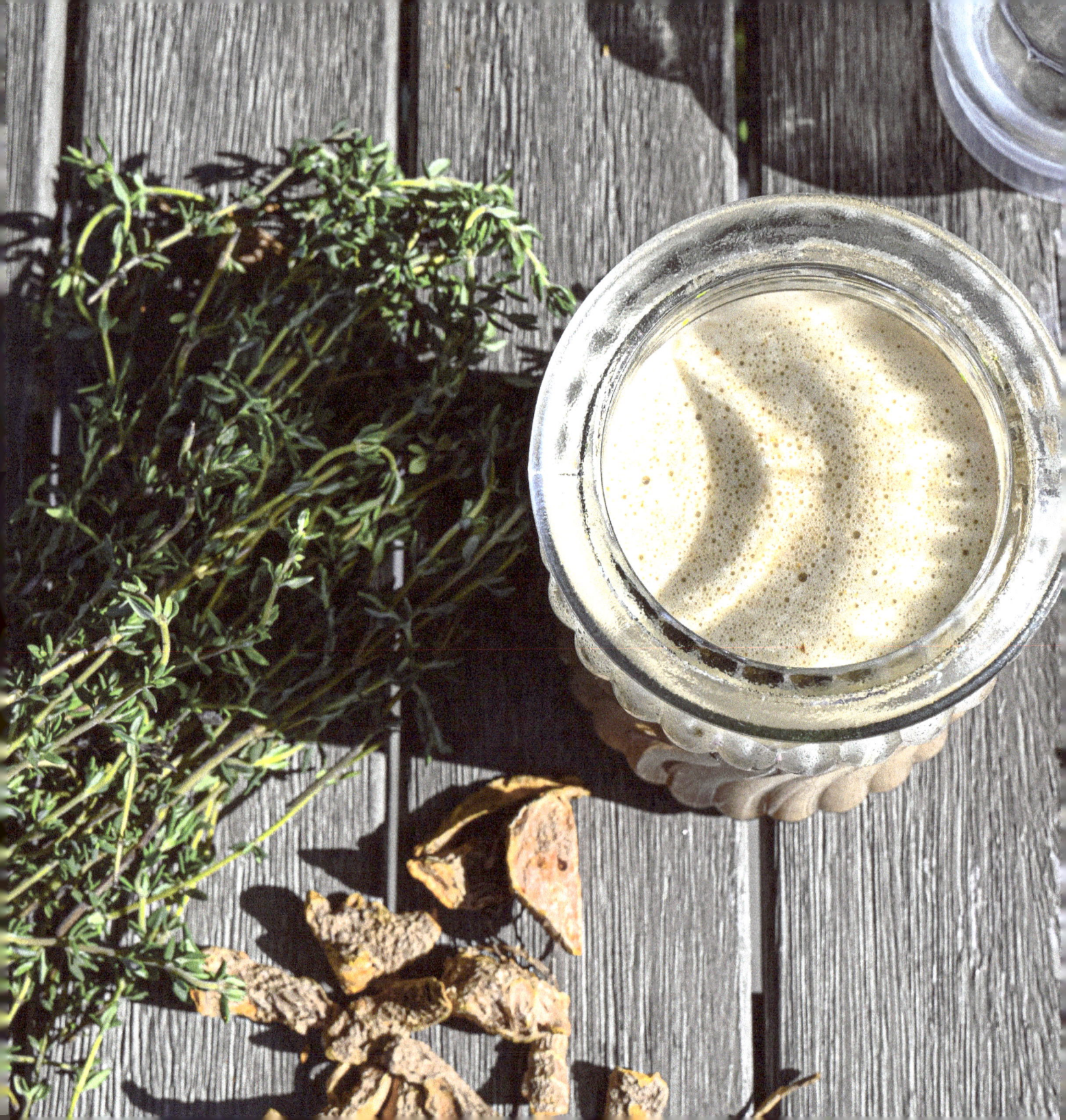

Thyme Seasoning

Serving size: 2

Equipment

- Glass bowl
- Whisk
- Mason jar

Ingredients

- 2 Tbsp lemon juice
- Juice of 2 clementines (yields ⅓ cup)
- 3 Tbsp tahini
- 1 Tbsp thyme, fresh and chopped
- 1 Tbsp basil, fresh and chopped
- 1 Tbsp olive oil
- 2 Tbsp coconut nectar
  +
- ⅛ tsp Guérance salt or Himalayan sea salt
- ⅛ tsp black pepper, ground

Instructions

1. In the glass bowl, whisk together all the ingredients except the salt and pepper.
2. Add salt and pepper and whisk again to combine.
3. Pour into mason jar and use immediately or store in refrigerator for up to 1 week.

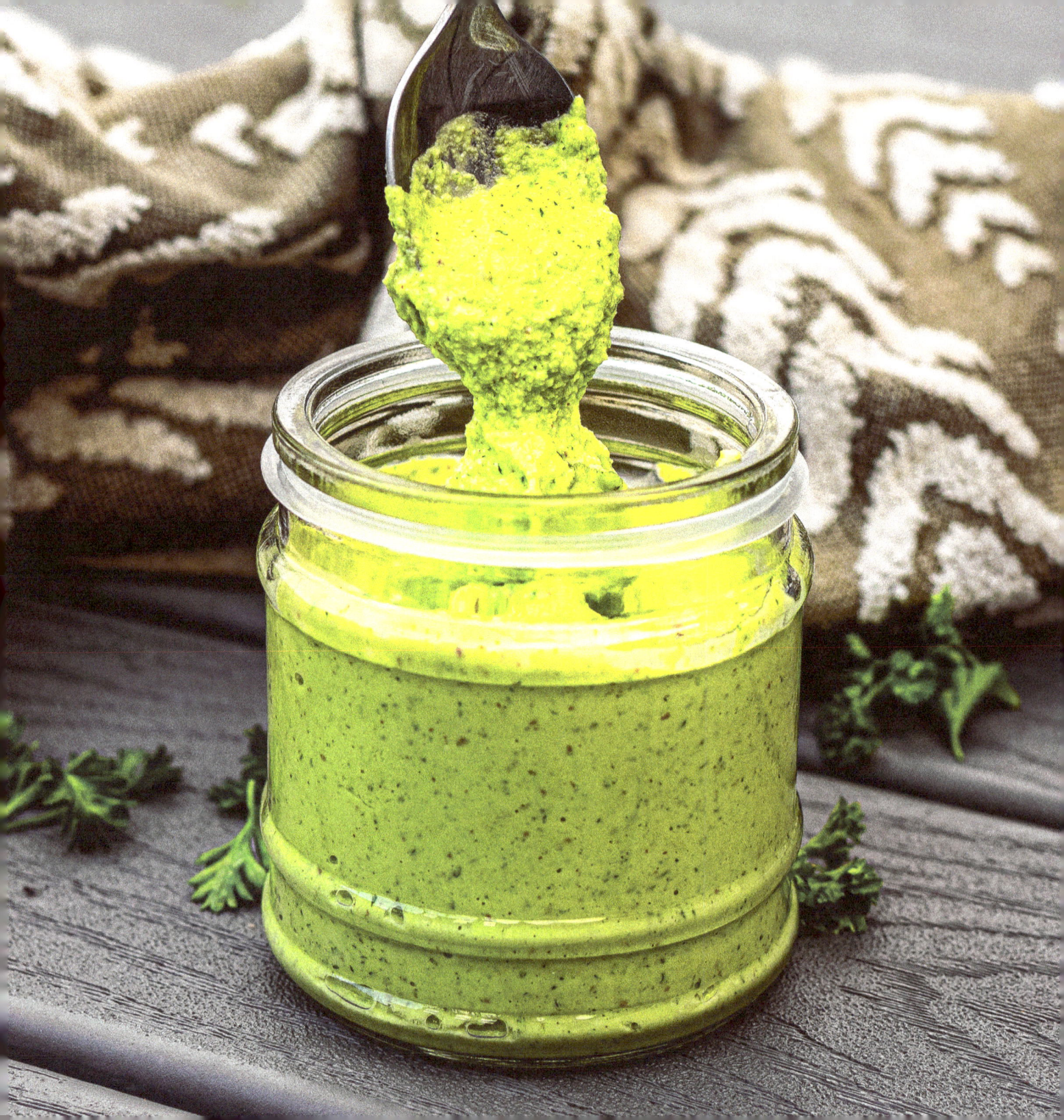

Raw Mamamia Pesto

Serving size: 5

Equipment
- High-speed blender
- Mason jar

Ingredients
- 1 cup parsley, fresh
- 1 Tbsp coriander, fresh
- ½ cup Brazil nuts, raw
- ½ cup cashews, soaked for 2 hours and rinsed
- ½ Tbsp lemon juice
- ⅛ tsp Himalayan sea salt
- ½ cup olive oil
- ½ cup water, filtered (*Quinton or Spring water*)

Instructions
1. Blend all ingredients.
2. Pour into mason jar.
3. Keep up to 5 days in refrigerator.

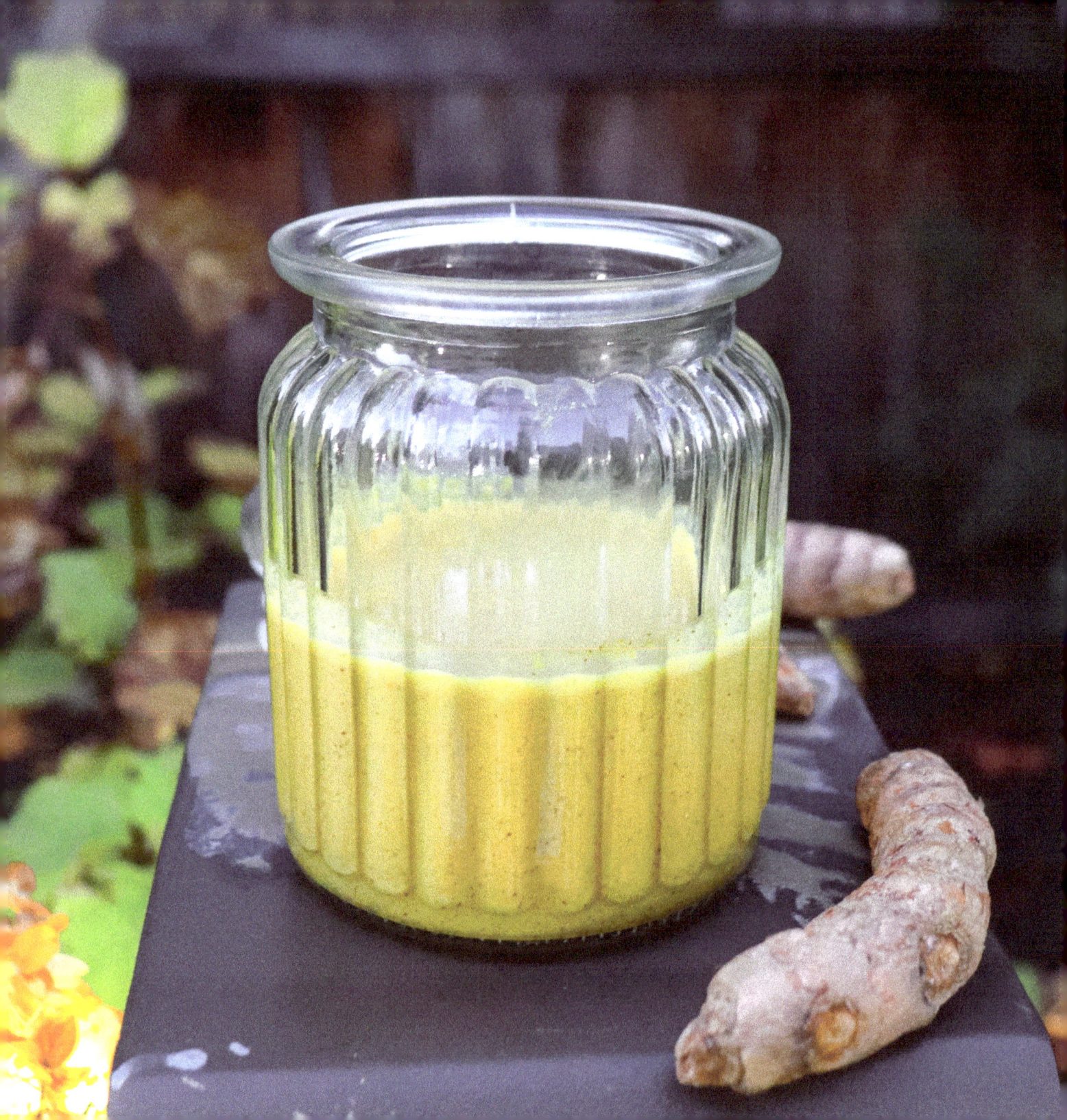

Turmeric Mixture

Serving size: 8

Equipment
- Mason jar or shallow container
- Knife
- Spoon
- High-speed blender

Ingredients
- ¼ cup almond butter
- ½ cup water, filtered
- 1 Tbsp lemon juice
- 1 Tbsp tahini
- 1 clove
- 2 Tbsp coconut nectar
- 1 tsp ground turmeric
- ¼ tsp Himalayan sea salt
- ⅛ tsp black pepper, ground.

Instructions
1. Add all ingredients to high-speed blender and blend until smooth.
2. Pour into mason jar.
3. Store in refrigerator for up to 7 days.

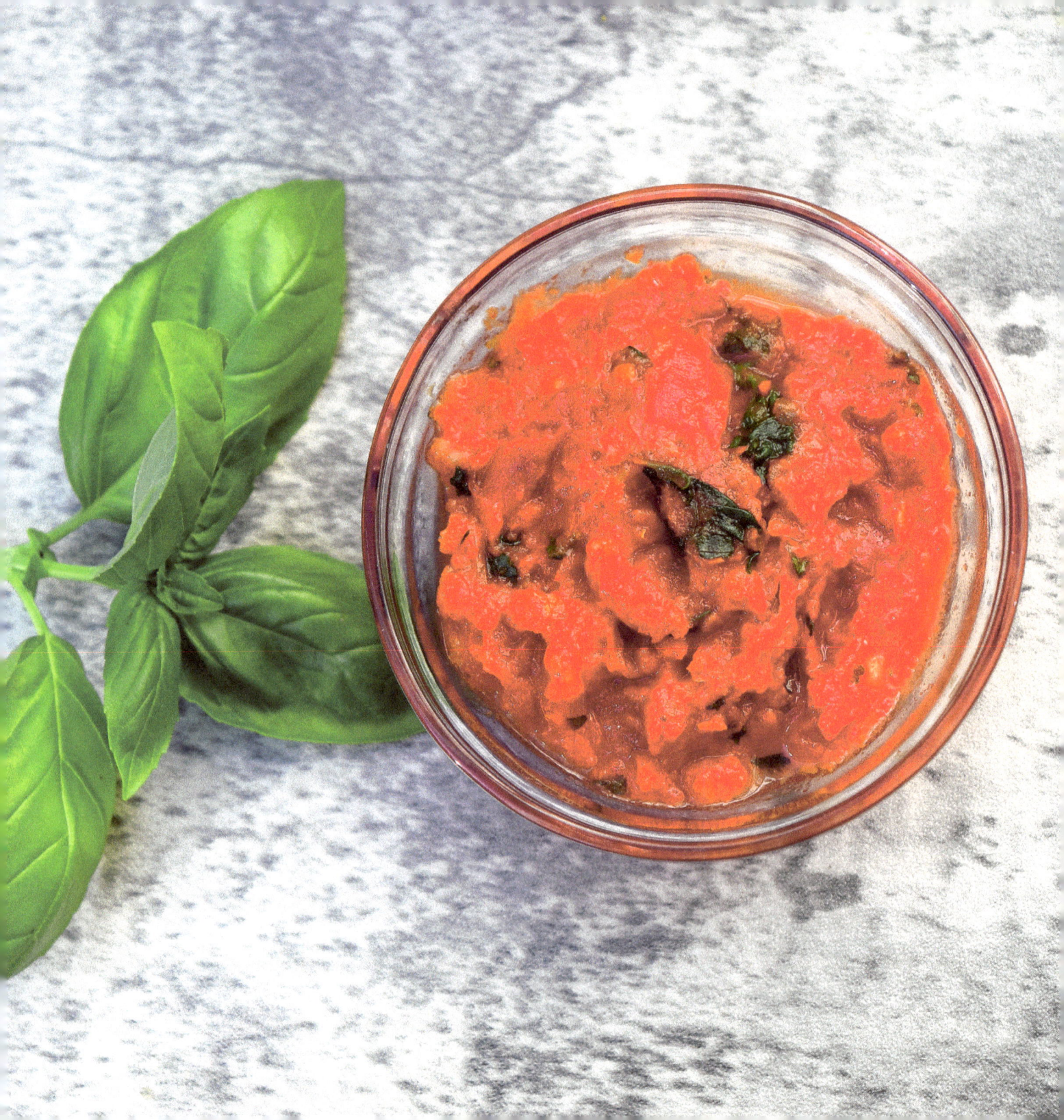

Basil Tomato Sauce

Serving size: 5

Equipment
- Shallow container
- High-speed blender

Ingredients
- ½ cup sun-dried tomatoes, soaked in ½ cup filtered water for a minimum of 4 hours
  +
- ½ cup tomatoes, de-seeded (about 2 tomatoes)
- 2 garlic cloves, minced
- ½ Tbsp thyme, fresh
- 2 Tbsp chiffonade basil
- 1 tsp herbes de Provence
- 1 Tbsp olive oil
- ¼ tsp Himalayan sea salt, to taste
- ⅛ tsp black pepper, ground

Instructions
1. Using a high-speed blender, blend the soaked sun-dried tomatoes with ¼ of the water it was soaked in.
2. Add remaining ingredients to previous mixture in blender and pulse a little bit (we want the final mixture to look chunky, not completely smooth).

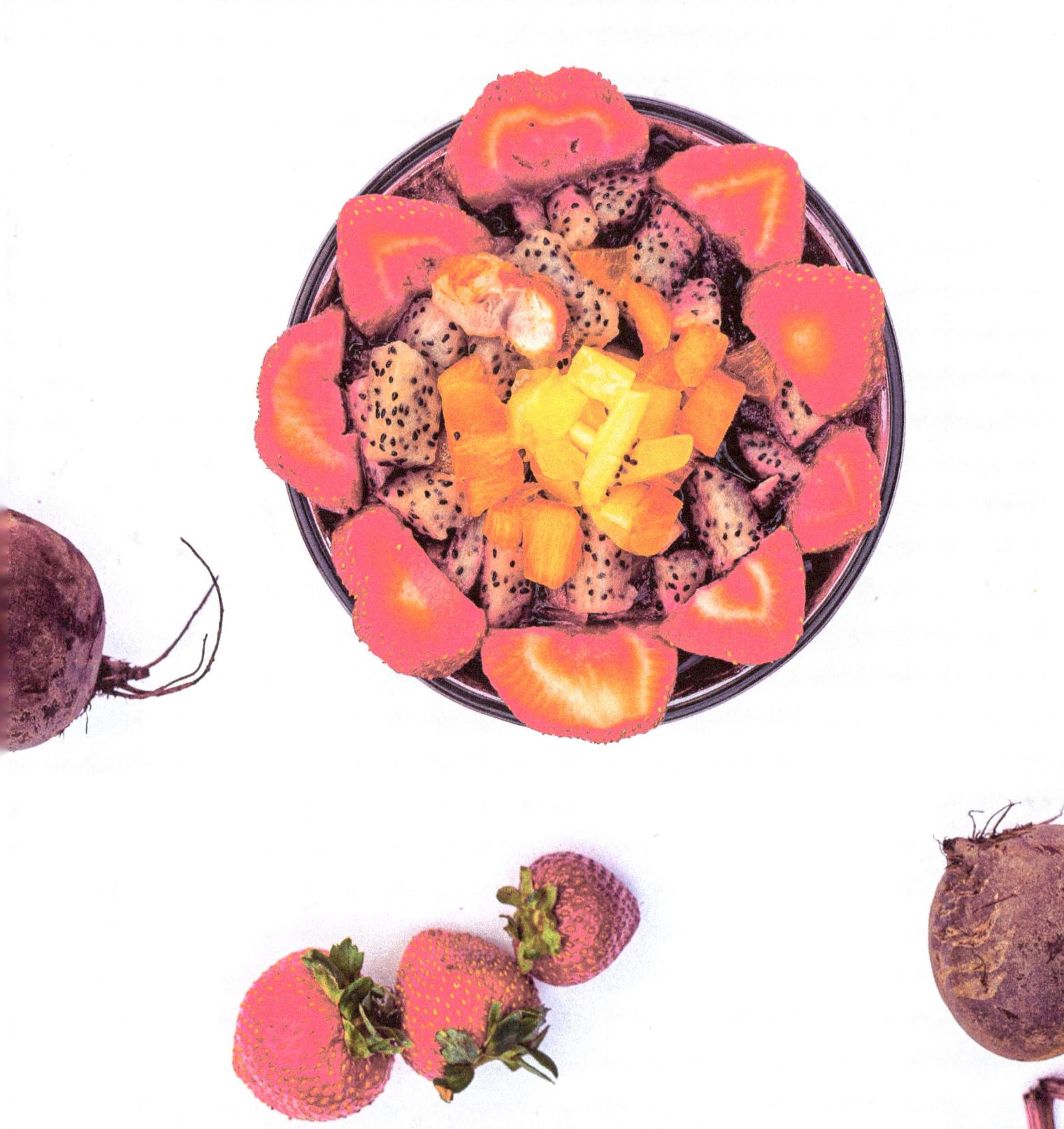

VI
FRUIT-BASED RECIPES

Unleash your creativity with the different textures and techniques of these fruit recipes.

Fruits should be considered as a separate meal and not as a dessert. We humans are great fruitarians! Ideally, we should have 40–60% fresh fruit and 20% dried fruits as part of our diet.

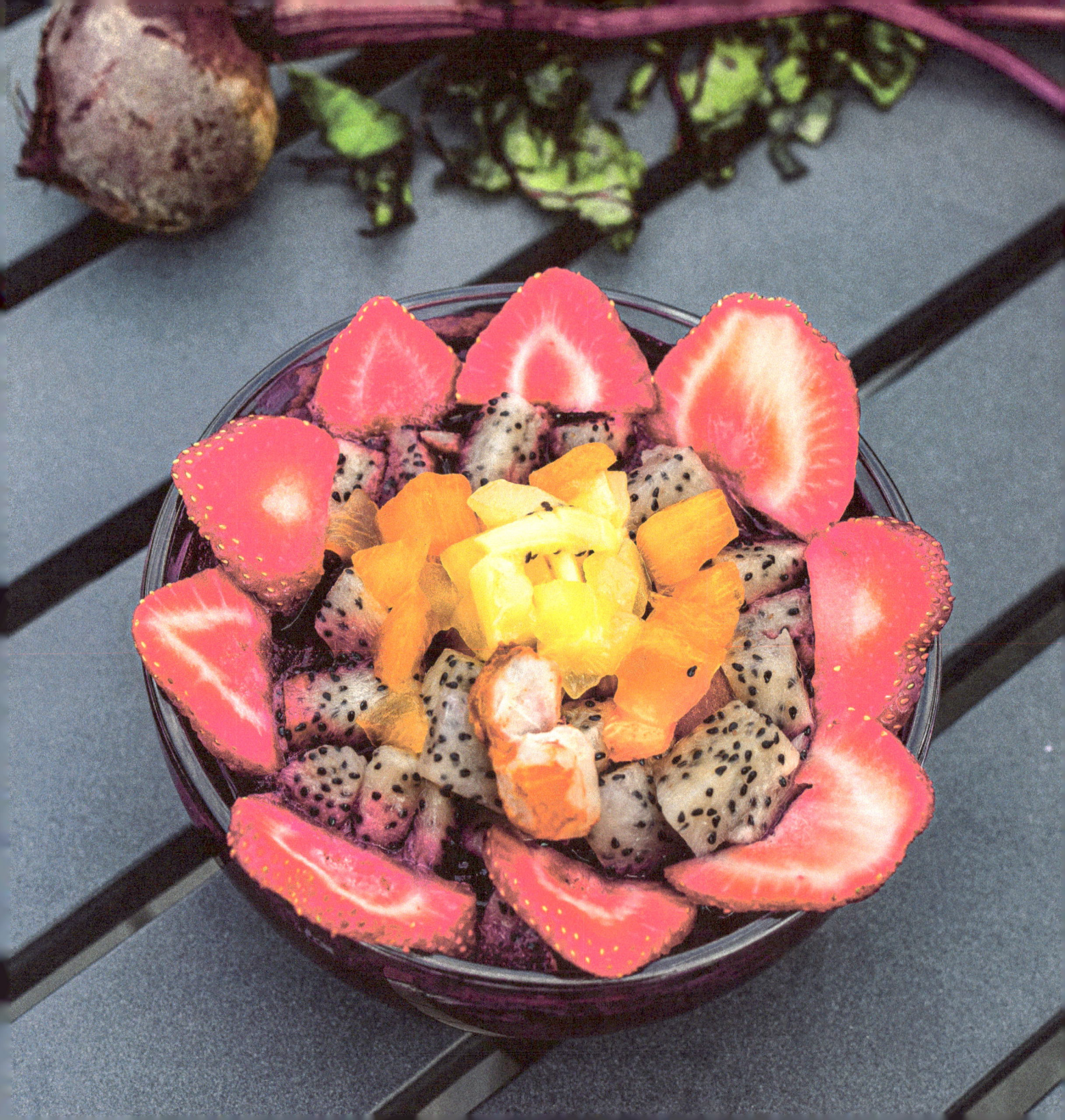

Exotic Mangosteen & Dragon Fruit Salad

Serving size: 1

Equipment
- Bowl
- Spoon

Ingredients
- 1 cup beet juice, freshly extracted using a juice extractor
  (2 large beets will yield 1 cup beet juice)
  +
- ½ dragon fruit, diced
- 1 mangosteen, peeled
- 1 apple, diced
- 3 fresh strawberries, finely sliced
- 1 kiwi, diced
- 1 persimmon, diced

Instructions
1. Pour beet juice into a bowl.
2. Add cut fruits to beet juice bowl.
3. Use the strawberries to decorate around the bowl.
4. Eat immediately or chill for 15 minutes in refrigerator.
5. Store in refrigerator for up to 2 days.

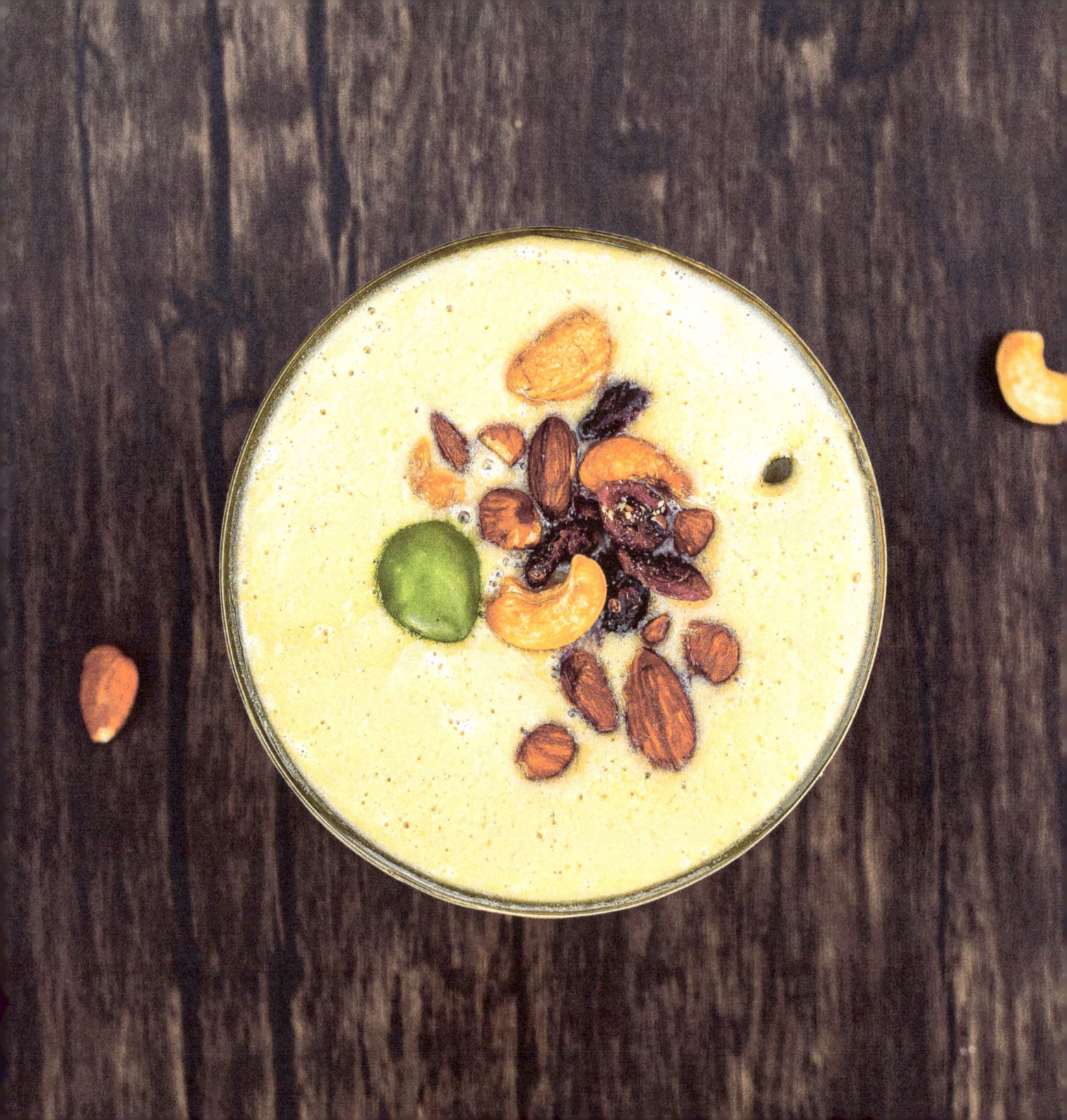

Almond Grape Frappé

Serving size: 2

Ingredients

- 1 cup raw almonds, soaked for 8 hours overnight and dehydrated
- 1 cup water
+
- ½ cup mango, frozen
- ¼ cup coconut nectar
+
- ½ cup grapes
- ¼ cup mixed nuts, dried raisins and cherries

Instructions

1. Blend almonds and water.
2. Using a nut milk bag, filter to get almond milk.
3. Discard the pulp or save in refrigerator for future use.
4. Return almond milk to cleaned blender.
5. Add frozen mangoes and coconut nectar.
6. Blend until smooth and pour into a smoothie bowl.
7. Add the grapes.
8. Top with nuts of your choice (*optional*).
9. Serve and eat immediately or store for 24 hours in refrigerator.

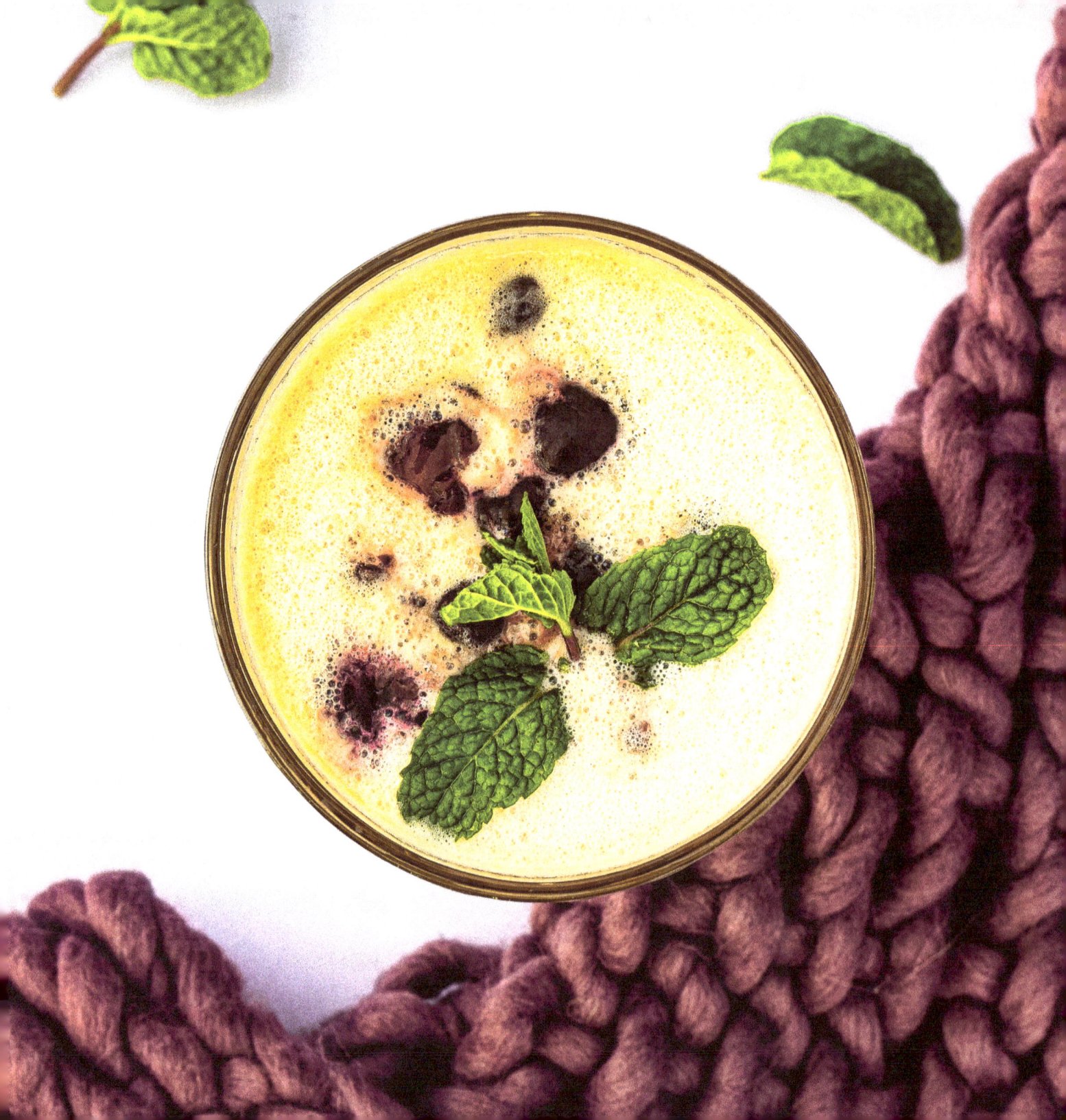

Pineapple Cherry Delish

Serving size: 2

Equipment

- 2 smoothie cups
- High-speed blender
- Spoon
- Nut milk bag

Ingredients

- 1 cup raw almonds, soaked for 8 hours or overnight and dehydrated
- 1 cup water

  +
- ½ cup pineapple, frozen
- ¼ cup agave nectar or coconut nectar

  +
- ½ cup organic fresh cherries, halved
- 4–6 fresh mint leaves

Instructions

1. Blend almonds and water.
2. Using a nut milk bag, filter to get almond milk.
3. Discard the pulp or save in refrigerator for future use.
4. Return almond milk to cleaned blender.
5. Add frozen pineapple and agave nectar.
6. Blend until smooth.
7. Pour half into a cup.
8. Add cherries.
9. Decorate with fresh mint leaf.
10. Repeat the same with the 2nd smoothie cup.
11. Serve and eat with a spoon.

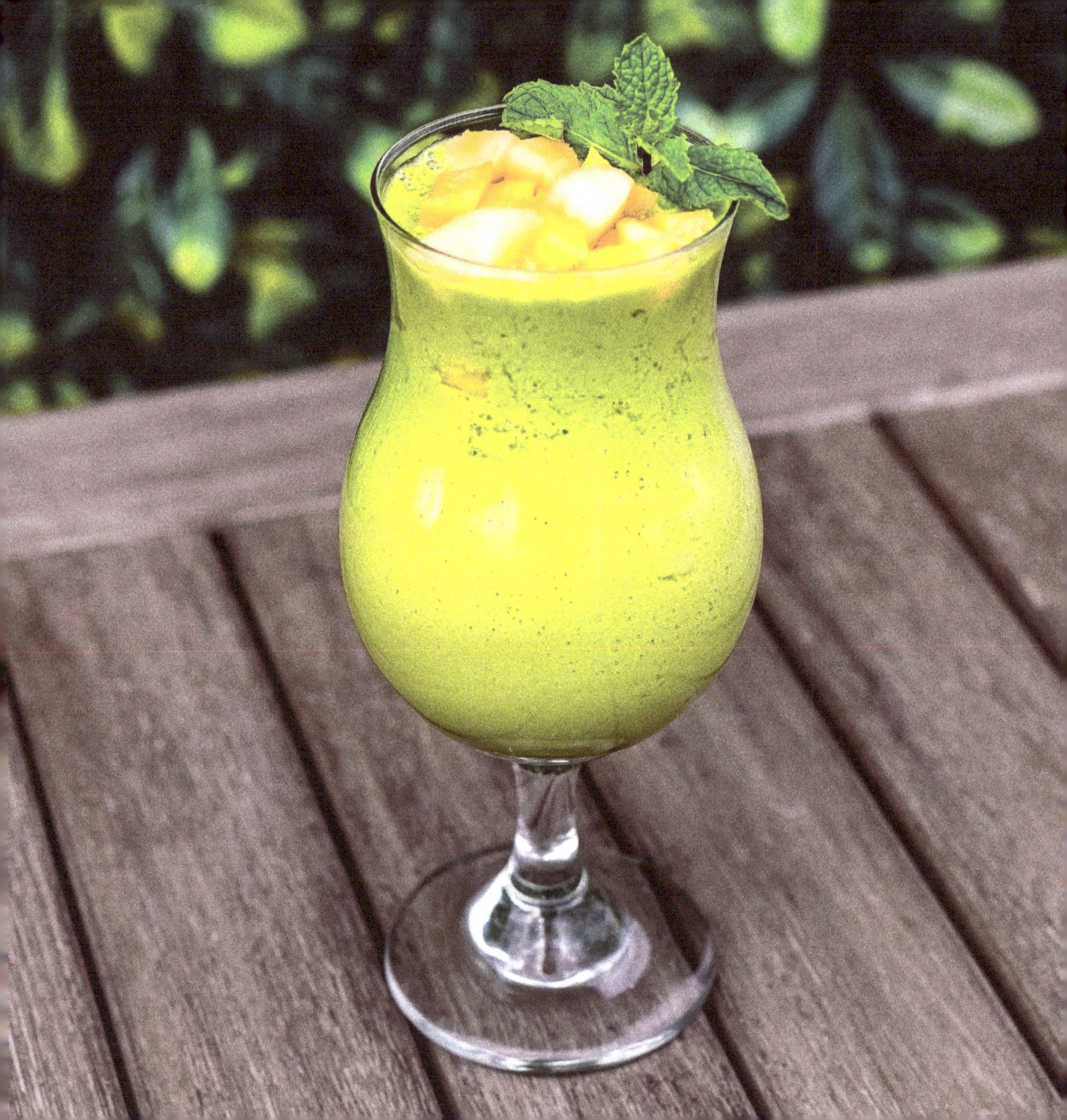

Apple Spinach Mix

Serving size: 1

Equipment

- Bowl
- High-speed blender
- Nut milk bag

Ingredients

- 1 cup raw almonds, soaked for 8 hours or overnight and dehydrated
- 1 cup water
  +
- ½ cup mangoes, frozen
- ¼ cup organic spinach, raw
- ¼ cup coconut nectar
  +
- 1 Tbsp organic apples
- ¼ cup mangoes, fresh

Decoration

- ½ fresh mint leaf

Instructions

1. Blend almonds and water.
2. Using nut milk bag, filter to get almond milk.
3. Return almond milk to cleaned blender.
4. Add frozen mangoes, spinach and coconut nectar.
5. Blend until smooth.
6. Pour into a bowl.
7. Add apples and mangoes.
8. Decorate with the fresh mint leaf.
9. Serve immediately or store for up to 3 days in refrigerator.

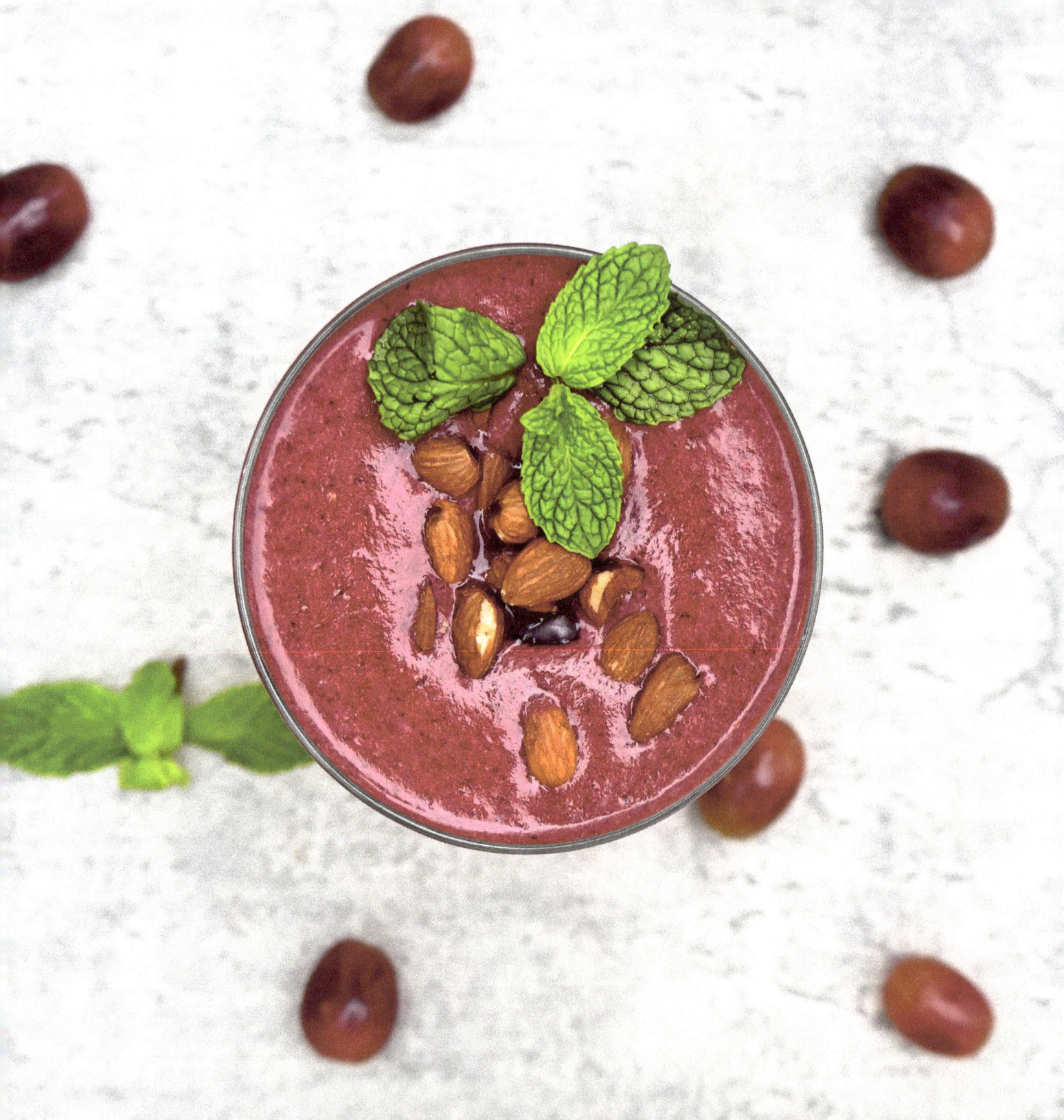

Mango Fruit Salad

Serving size: 1

Equipment
- High-speed blender
- Cup

Ingredients
- ½ cup almond milk (obtained from blending ½ cup raw almonds, soaked for 8 hours and dehydrated with ½ cup water. Filter with nut milk bag.)
- ½ cup mangoes, fresh
- ½ cup mixed berries, frozen
- 2 Tbsp coconut nectar

Instructions
1. Add all ingredients to blender and blend until smooth.
2. Decorate with fresh fruits of your choice.
3. Serve immediately in a cup or store in the refrigerator for 24 hours.

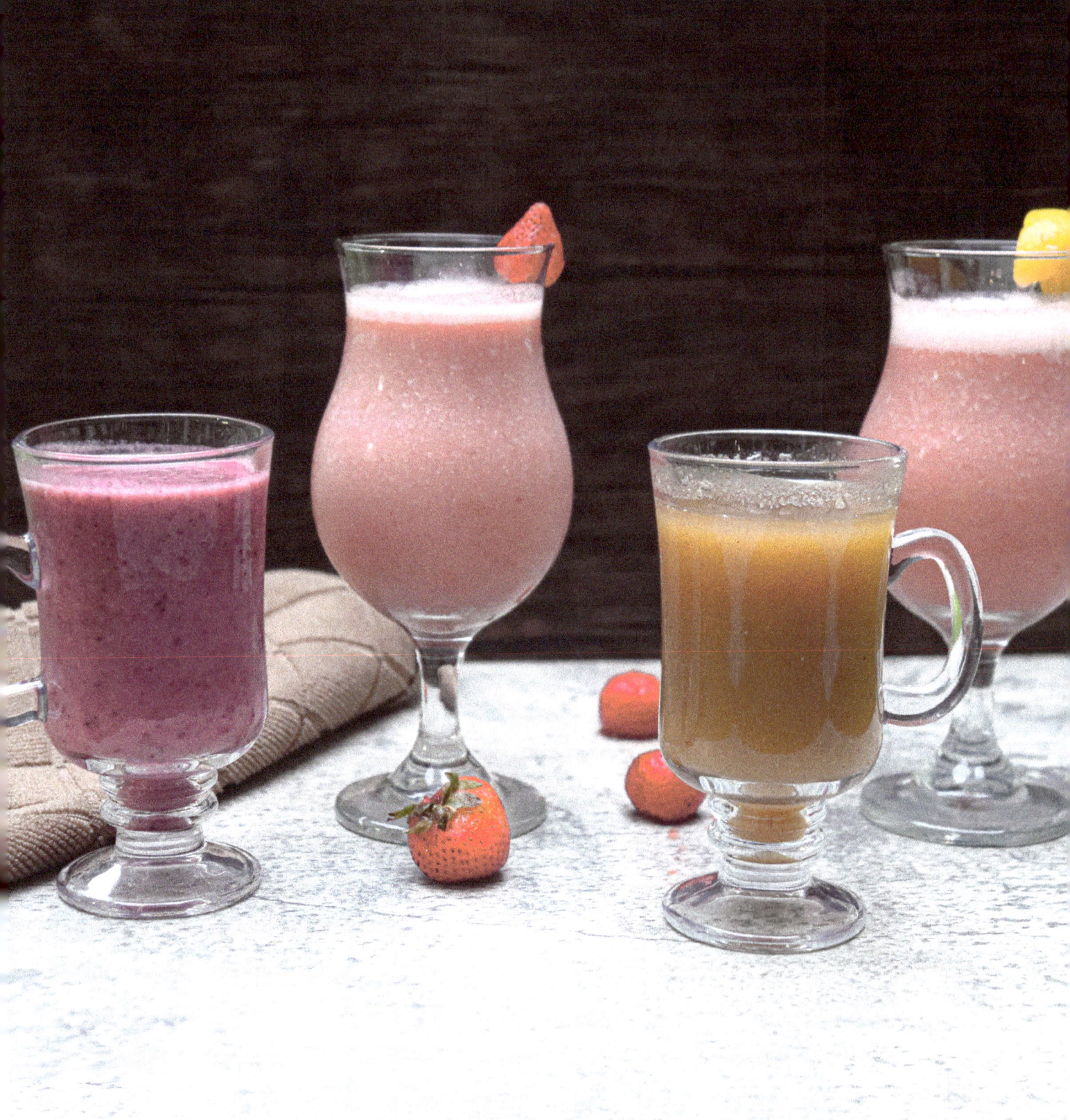

VII
SMOOTHIES

There's nothing like a good fruit smoothie in the morning to fill you with energy and welcome the beautiful day that is offered to you.

Drinking smoothies is a great way to nourish the body with the nutrients it needs. It is often confused with juicing, which is quite different. While juicing takes out the pulp from the recipe for easy absorption of the nutrients by the body, smoothies provide the flexibility of keeping the pulp in the recipe while exploring different Ingredients and textures.

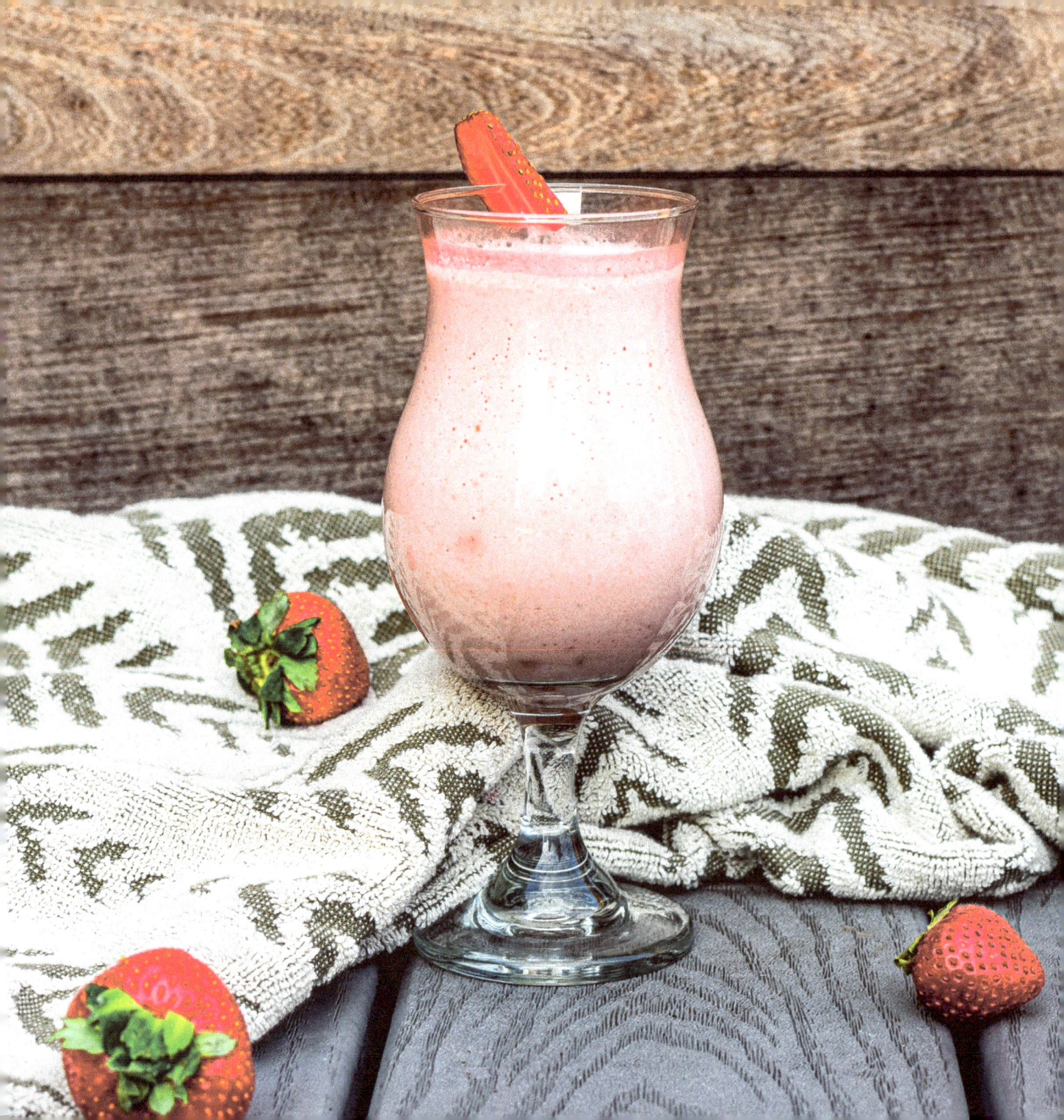

Strawberry Smoothie

Serving size: 1

Equipment

- Knife
- Bowl
- Spoon
- High-speed blender

Ingredients

- 9 strawberries, fresh
  +
- ½ cup almond milk (obtained from blending soaked and dehydrated almonds with water)
- 8 dates, dried
  +
- 1 strawberry for decoration

Instructions

1. Using a knife, cut strawberries into quarters. Set aside.
2. Add almond milk and dates to the blender and incorporate the quartered strawberries.
3. Blend until smooth.
4. Pour into bowl.
5. Garnish with the 1 remaining strawberry.
6. Consume immediately or store for 5 days in refrigerator.

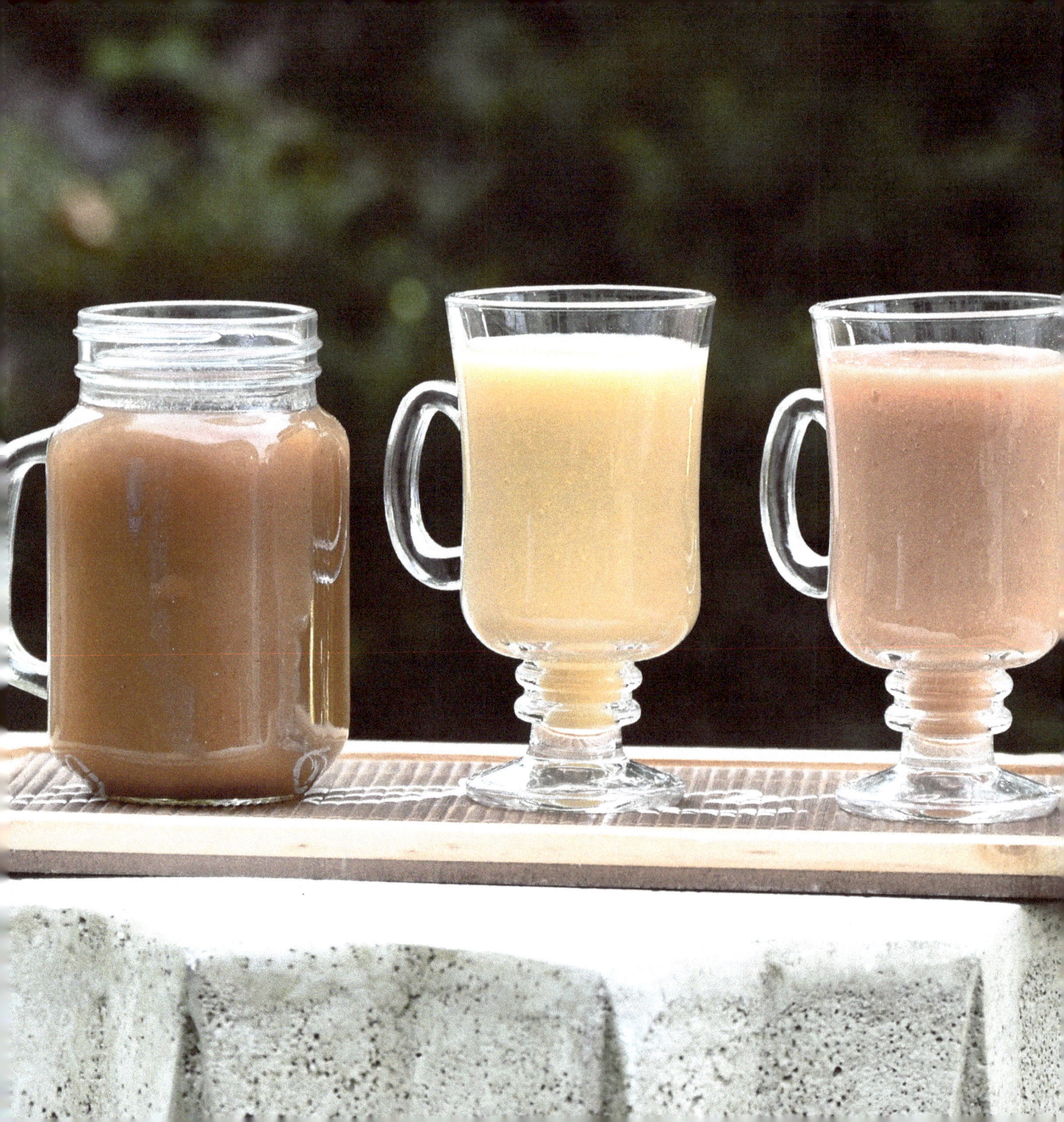

Guava, Pomegranate, Baobab

Serving size: 1 each

GUAVA NECTAR

Equipment

High-speed blender

Ingredients

- 1 cup water + 2 Tbsp water
- 4 Tbsp coconut nectar
- 1 cup guava fruit (no need to peel the skin)

Instructions

1. Add all ingredients to blender and blend until smooth.
2. Pour into a cup and enjoy or store in refrigerator for up to 1 week.

POMEGRANATE NECTAR

Equipment

High-speed blender

Ingredients

- 2 Tbsp pomegranate juice
- 2 pears
- 3 Tbsp coconut nectar

Instructions

1. Add all ingredients to high-speed blender and blend until smooth.
2. Pour into a cup and enjoy or store in refrigerator for up to 1 week.

BAOBAB NECTAR

Equipment

- Cup
- Whisk
- High-speed blender
- Pot

Ingredients

- ⅓ cup baobab powder
- ⅔ cup water
  +
- 2 cups water, filtered
- 4 Tbsp coconut nectar

Instructions

1. In glass bowl, mix baobab powder and ⅔ cup water using whisk.
2. Bring to a boil for 3 minutes at low temperature.
3. Remove from stove and let cool.
4. Add coconut nectar and whisk again.
5. Pour into a cup and enjoy or store in refrigerator for up to 1 week.

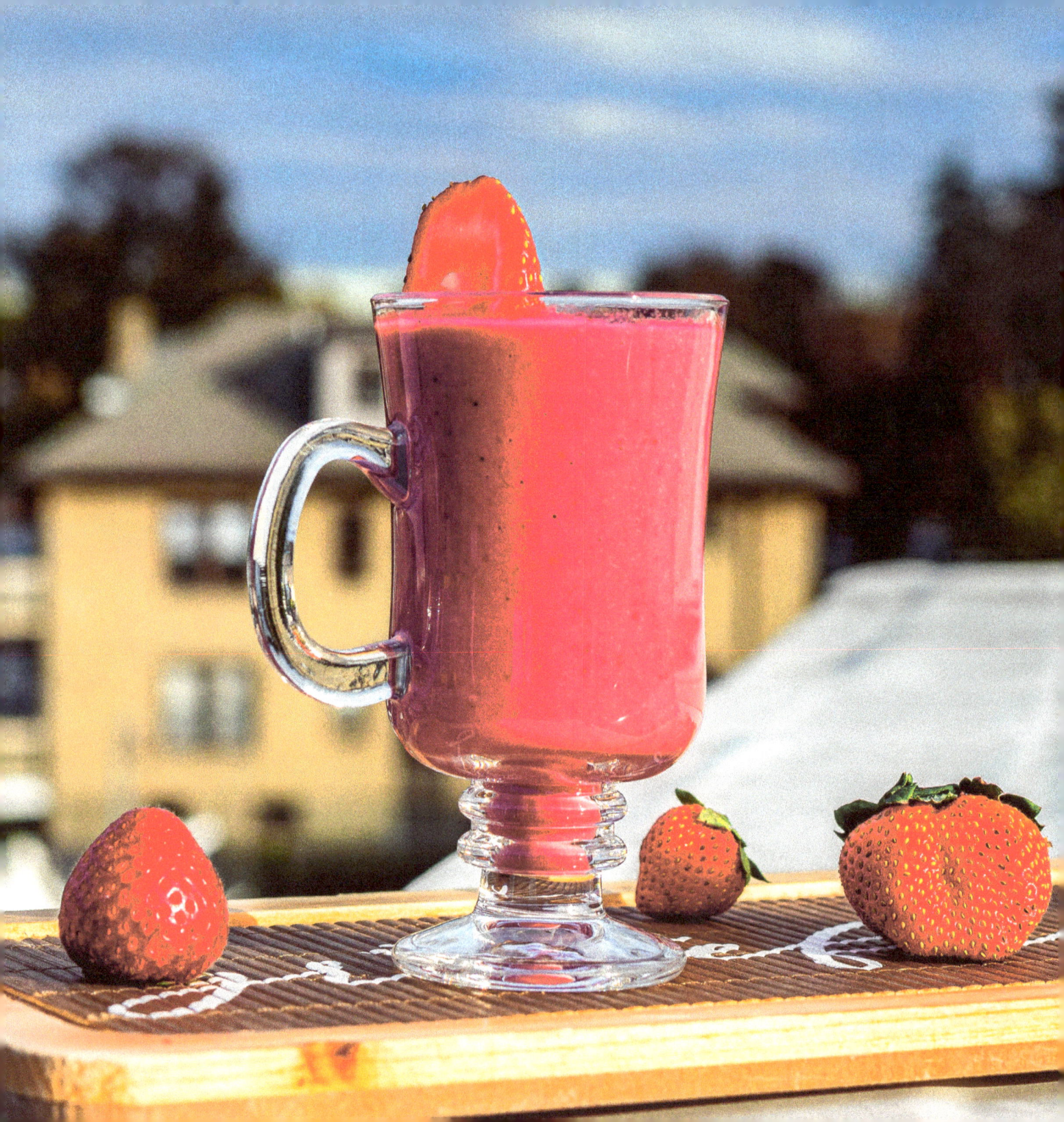

Coconut Berry Smoothie

Serving size: 1

Equipment
- High-speed blender
- Bowl

Coconut Milk Ingredients
- 3 cups water
- 1 cup coconut, shredded

Smoothie Ingredients
- ½ cup homemade coconut milk
- 1 cup berries, frozen (mix of blackberries, blueberries, strawberries)
- 2 Medjool dates, pitted (you can add more for more sweetness)
- 1 scoop acerola powder (vitamin c) or mesquite powder
- 1 Tbsp juice of a clementine
- *Optional*: 1 scoop of organic iron pure food powder

Filling Ingredients
- 1 cup organic grapes
- ½ cup organic peaches (*de-seeded*)

Topping Ingredients:
1 cup your favorite allergy-safe organic nuts and dried fruits (we have used almonds, walnuts, dried cherries, dried cranberries)

Instructions
1. Blend the coconut milk ingredients in high-speed blender and strain.
2. Set aside ½ cup coconut milk and store the remainder in refrigerator for 3–5 days.
3. Add all Smoothie ingredients to cleaned blender with the ½ cup coconut milk and blend until smooth.
4. Add peaches and grapes from Filling ingredients to a bowl.
5. Pour blended smoothie on top of the fruits.
6. Sprinkle with ingredients from Topping set. Enjoy!
7. Eat immediately or store in refrigerator up to 24 hours.

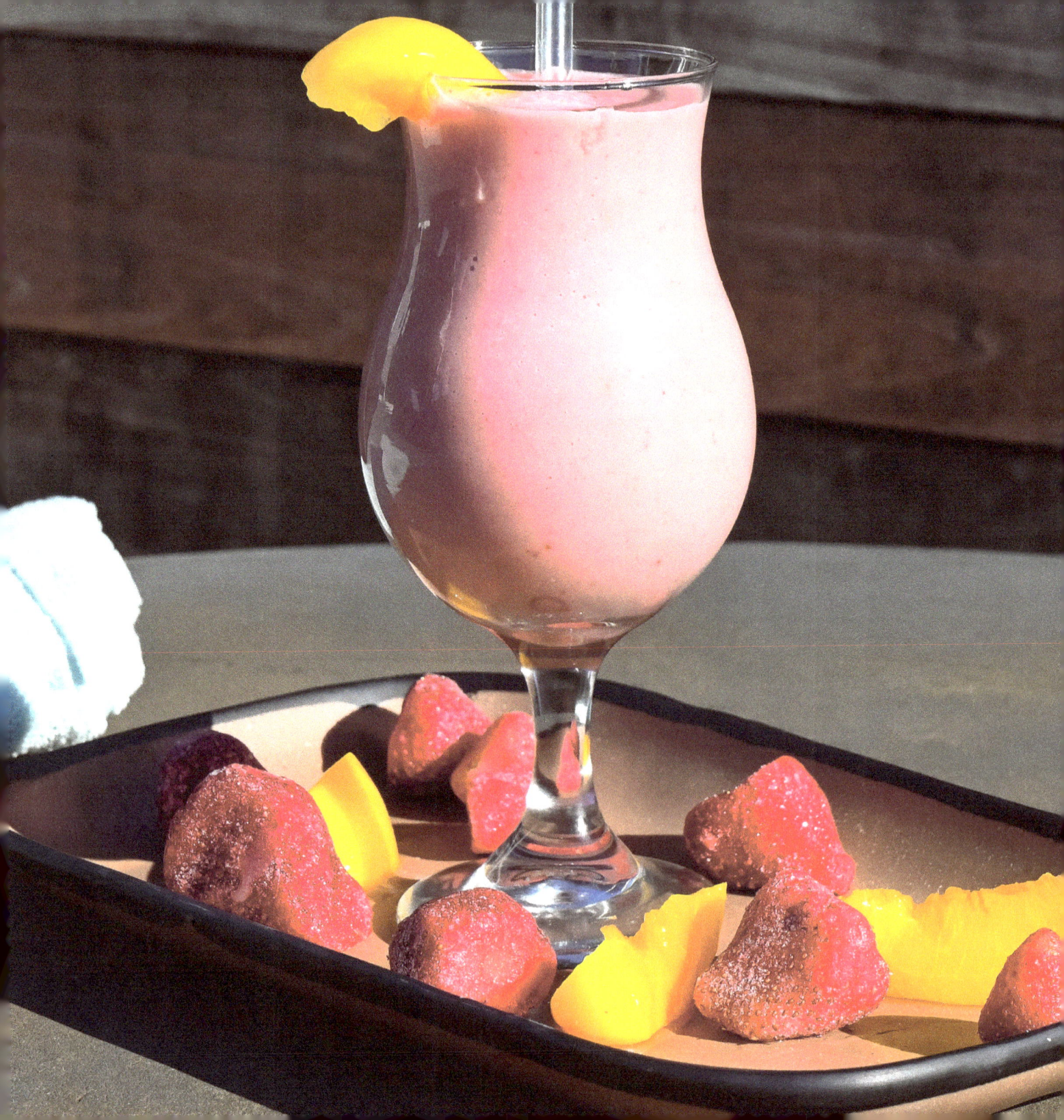

Peach Strawberry Smoothie

Serving size: 1

Equipment
- High-speed blender
- Bowl or cup

Ingredients
- 1 cup raw milk of your choice (coconut, almond milk, tiger nut milk, etc.)
- ½ cup peaches, frozen
- ½ cup strawberries, frozen
- ¼ cup agave nectar or any other sweetener of your choice

Topping Ingredients
Strawberries and peaches

Instructions
1. Add all ingredients to high-speed blender and blend until smooth.
2. Pour into a cup of your choice.
3. Decorate with strawberries and peaches.

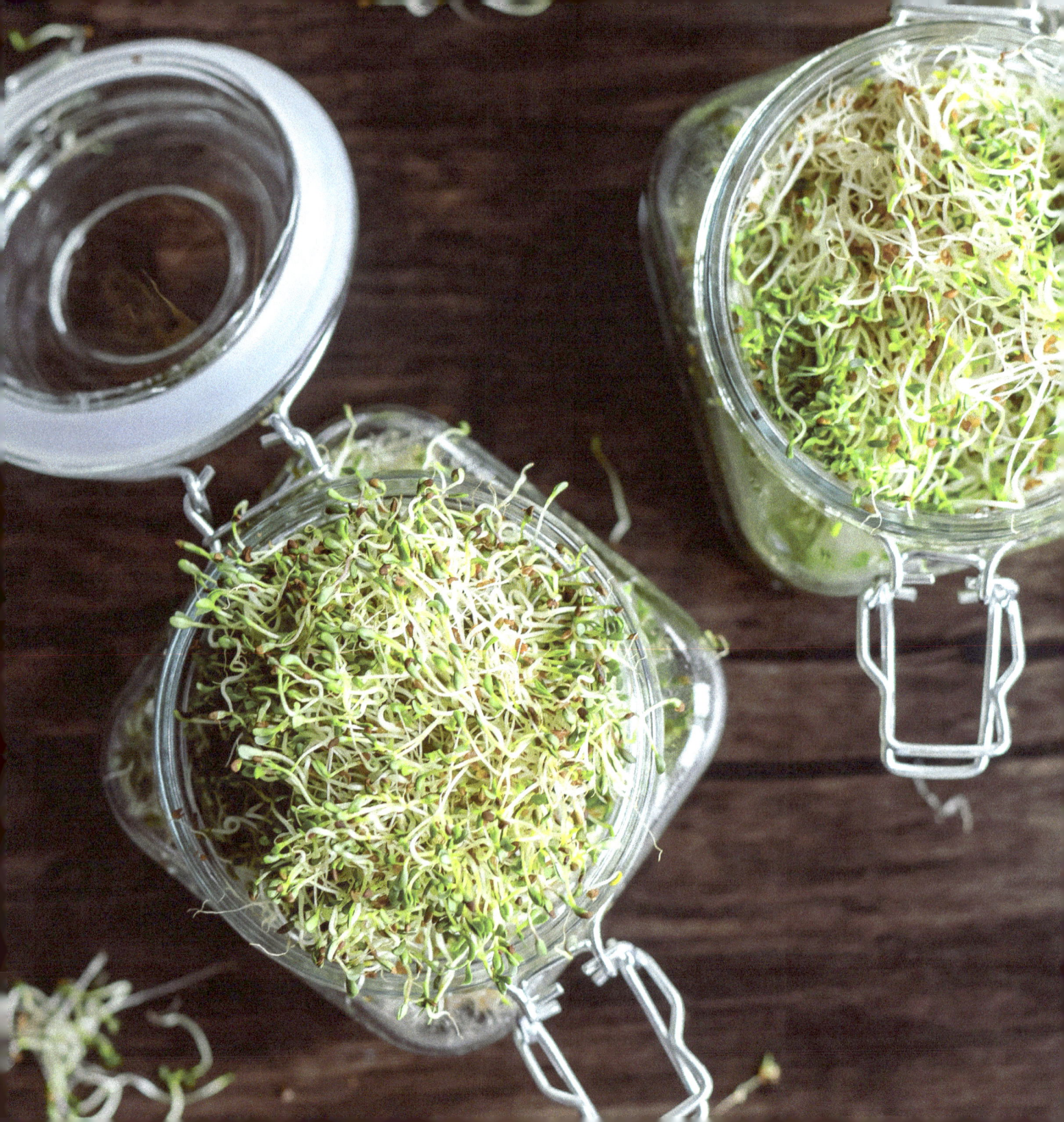

VIII
MAKE YOUR SPROUTED SEEDS & YOUNG SPROUTS

"Life Generates Life"

The secret of intrinsic vitality comes from a natural, raw and living diet. Sprouts and sprouted seeds are 10 to 100 times more concentrated than mature grains.

THE BENEFITS OF SPROUTS

"May your food be your only medicine," said Hippocrates (460 - 370 BC), who is recognized as the founding father of Western medicine. Indeed, the benefits of sprouts have been known since antiquity, especially in Asia (China) and Africa (Egypt).

Today, the cultivation and consumption of sprouts is booming. In addition to being part of a living and natural diet, several scientific studies have proven the health benefits of sprouts.

These studies show that sprouts contain an enriching concentration of antioxidants, enzymes, vitamins and minerals necessary for the proper functioning of the body.

SPROUTS IN DIET

Y.M. Lee and colleagues have shown that sprouts help strengthen the immune system. In one of the studies referenced in his book, Lee concluded that "increasing evidence suggests that peanut sprout root extract (PSRE) has anti-inflammatory activity." He also indicated that, "the sprouting process promotes significant changes in bioactive compounds that contain various types of phenolic compounds, many of which are antioxidants." Similarly, plant melatonin levels are high in shoots and plants. Melatonin is an endogenous natural antioxidant hormone that decreases with age. Low levels of melatonin are associated with several chronic diseases.

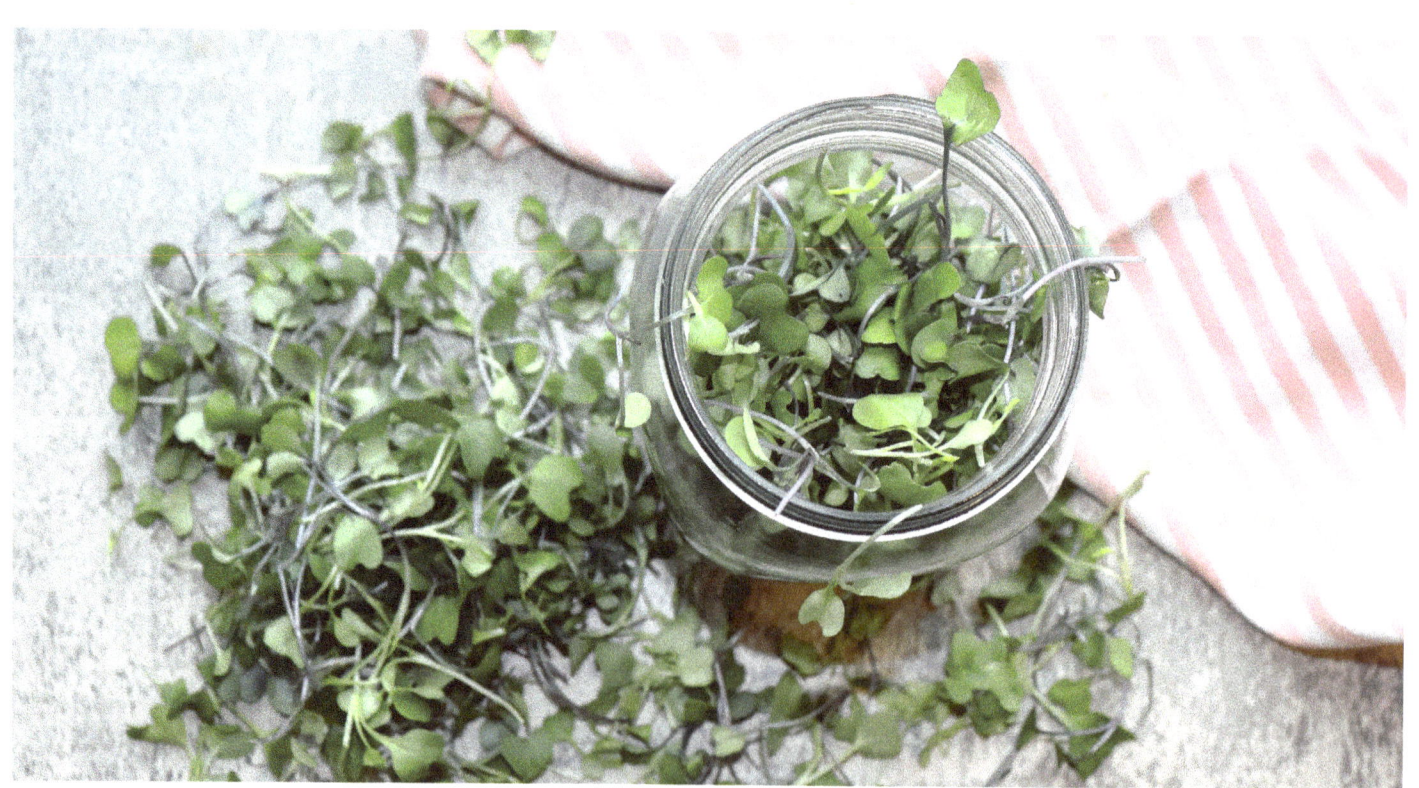

Sprouts, for the most part, are easy to grow and are usually ready for consumption after 5 to 7 days. Eating sprouts allows you to have fresh, crunchy, and most important, living products. They have a higher concentration of nutrients than traditional vegetables.

Micro-sprouts provide an additional plant source rich in bioactive components, glucosinolates and organic compounds with antioxidant and anti- carcinogenic properties. (Marton et al., 2010; Moreno et al., 2006).

USE OF RAW JUICES (INCLUDING SPROUTS)

Researchers in biology and nutrition around the world have demonstrated that a diet consisting specifically of raw foods (sprouts, raw fruits and vegetables) from organic crops opposes the action of cancer-causing substances. They are even effective in mitigating diseases that are already apparent. Dr. Virginia Livingston, immunotherapy specialist and cancer expert in the United States, recommends fresh and raw juices (sprouts, cabbage, cucumber, spinach, tomato, red beetroot, apple, orange and carrot) up to 1 liter per day to cancer patients.

IMPACT OF MICRO SPROUTS ON HEALTH

Many vitamins, amino acids and minerals can be manufactured (synthesized) in a laboratory. Even if they are consumed in specific quantities, they offer little value because they do not possess the vitality available in natural, raw, fresh and organic foods. "Micro-gardens" offer a variety of micro-shoots of high quality, fresh, specific, natural and organic food. These unprocessed shoots are a real treasure of vitality. They are easily digested, rich in chlorophyll and bring essential bioenergy that increases the vitality of those who ingest them regularly. Ideally, micro-sprouts should be grown on soil with osmosis-filtered water (pure water that is free of chlorine, lead, drug residues, mercury and pesticides).

References

Y.M. Lee et al., 2019. *Treatment with Peanut Sprout Root Extract Alleviates Inflammation in a Lipopolysaccharide–Stimulated Mouse Macrophage Cell Line by Inhibiting the MAPK Signaling Pathway.*

Aguilera et al., 2016. *Intake of bean sprouts influences melatonin and antioxidant capacity biomarker levels in rats.*

Màrton, M.; Màndoki, Z.; Csapó-Kiss, Z.; Csapó, J. *The role of sprouts in human nutrition. A review.* Acta Universitatis *Sapientiae Alimentaria* 2010, 3, 81–117.

Moreno, D.A.; Carvajal, M.; López-Berenguer, C.; García-Viguera, C. *Chemical and biological characterization of nutraceutical compounds of broccoli.*

J. Pharm. Biomed. Anal. 2006, 41, 1508– 1522.

Livingston, Virginia and Wheeler, Owen, *Food Alive.* The Livingston Wheeler Medical clinic. San Diego, 1977.

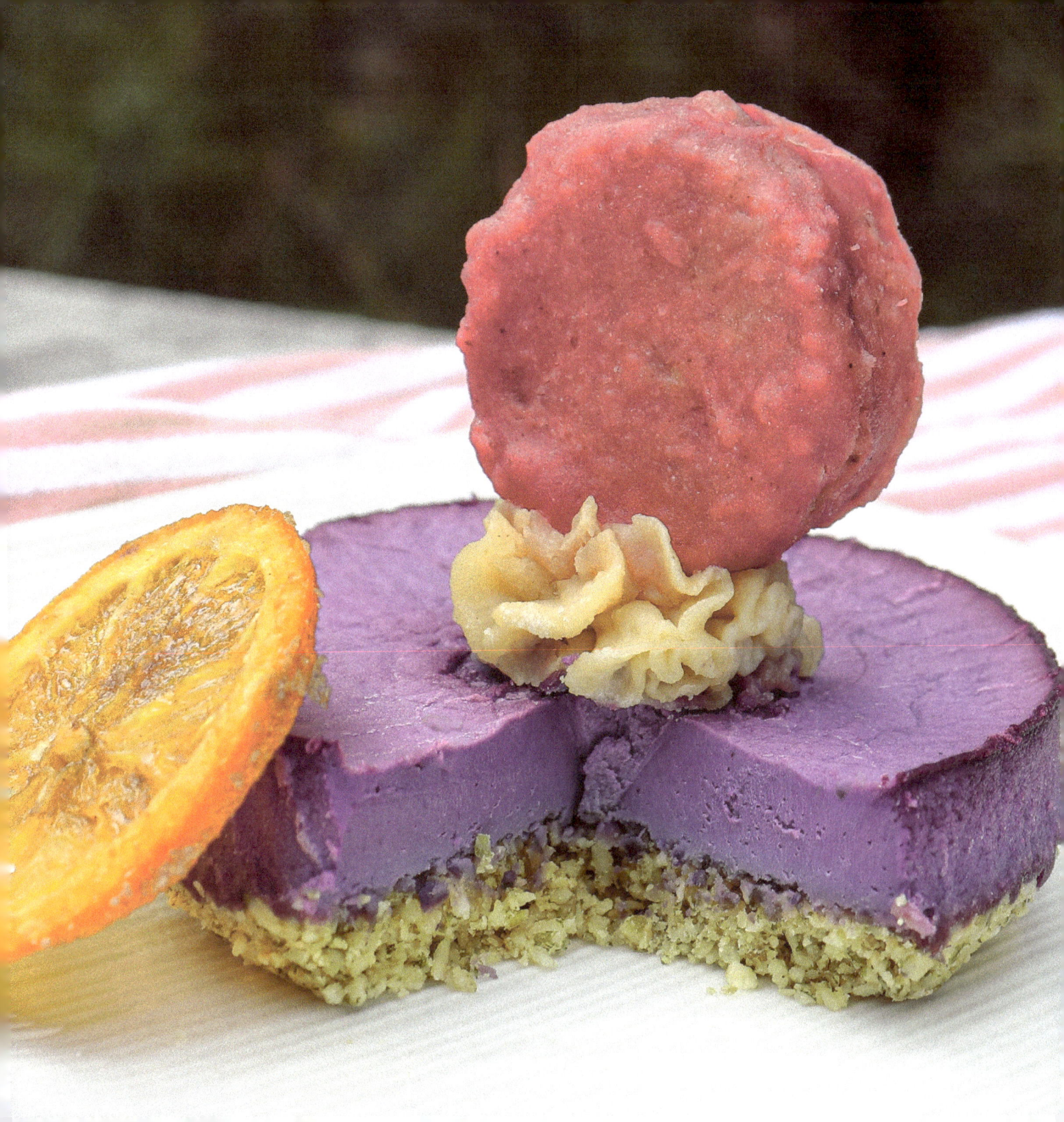

IX
RAW PLANT-BASED DESSERTS

The pleasure of eating sweet healthy flavors

Raw plant-based desserts are delicious and beautiful. Making these desserts from scratch (from the Ingredients to the final product) will unleash your creativity and desire to learn more as you master the art of processing, blending, dehydrating and much more.

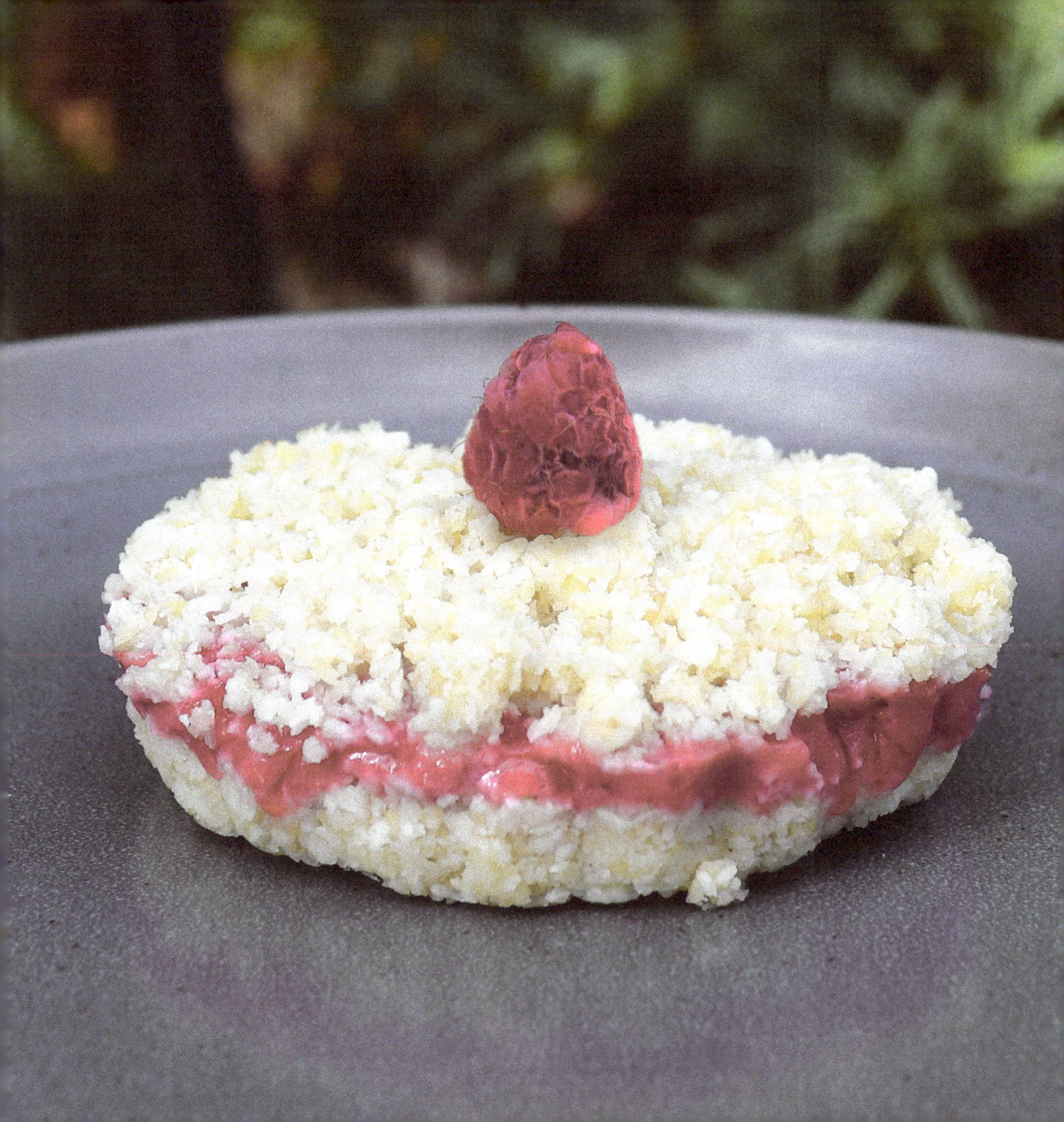

Raspberry Cake with Coconut

Serving size: 1

Equipment
- Food processor
- 4-inch round cake mold with pusher (3)
- High-speed blender
- Spatula

Bar Ingredients
- 2 cups coconut, shredded and dried
- ½ cup raw cashews, soaked for 2 hours, rinsed and dehydrated
- ¼ cup coconut nectar
- 2 drops vanilla essence

Raspberry Jam Ingredients
- 1½ cups raspberries
- ½ cup agave nectar

Instructions
1. Process all ingredients for the bars in food processor until you get a texture that looks like a crumble.
2. Take about ¾ of white crumble texture and press firmly into the cake ring mold using the cake ring mold pusher.
3. Put in freezer for about 10 minutes for it to start firming up.
4. Add all raspberry jam ingredients to high-speed blender using a spatula and blend until you get a smooth texture.
5. Remove base from freezer.
6. Add jam mixture on top of bars.
7. Sprinkle remaining crumble texture on top of the bars.
8. Freeze again for about 10 minutes.
9. Remove from freezer and serve immediately.
10. Store for up to 3 days in refrigerator.

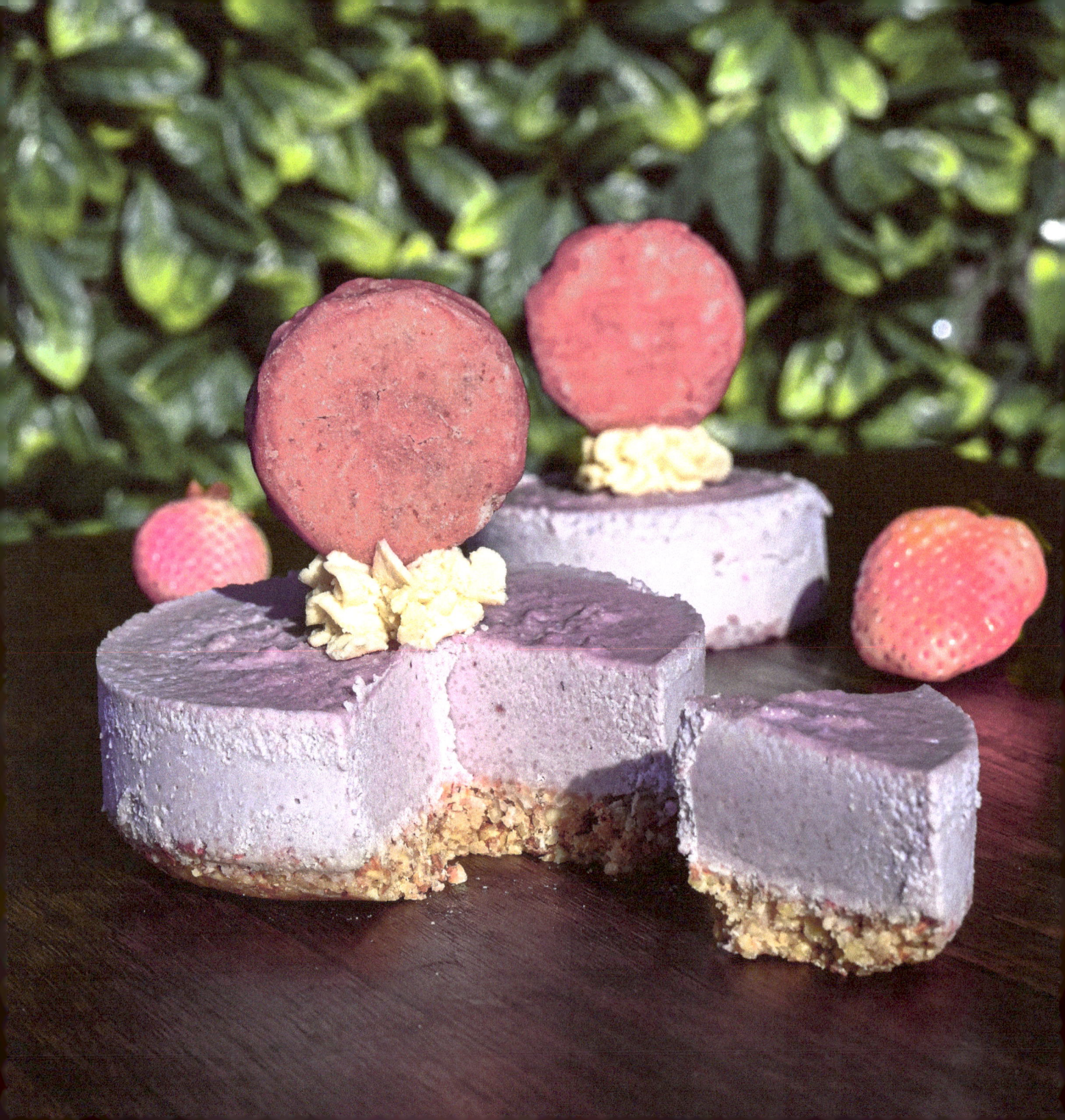

Hibiscus Macaron Cheesecake

Serving size: 2 small cheesecakes

Equipment

- High-speed blender
- Food processor
- Two 4-inch springform pans
- Cutting board
- Plastic wrap
- Pastry bag
- Spoon
- Dehydrator
- 1M piping tip
- 1 piping bag
- little cookie cutter (round shape and 3 inches wide)
- Glass bowl
- Parchment paper

Pumpkin Seed Crust Ingredients

- ½ cup pumpkin seeds
- ½ cup medium shredded coconut
- 2 Tbsp Lakanto monkfruit sweetener, powdered
- ½ Tbsp mesquite powder
- 1 Tbsp orange juice

  +
- 1 Tbsp coconut oil
- 3 drops strawberry essence, alcohol-free
- 3 drops vanilla essence, alcohol-free

Pumpkin Seed Crust Instructions

1. Before you start, bring the Lakanto to powder by blending it for a few seconds in high-speed blender. Set aside.
2. Process the pumpkin seed crust ingredients *(except coconut oil and essences)* in food processor until mixture forms a flour. If the texture is a little bit grainy after processing, that's fine.
3. Add coconut oil and strawberry and vanilla essences until batter starts sticking together.
4. Place two 4-inch springform pans on a cutting board.
5. Line the pans with plastic wrap.
6. Press mixture into bottom of the pans. Use the back of a spoon to smooth out crust.
7. Set in freezer while making the filling.

Hibiscus Filling Ingredients

- ½ cup hibiscus flower
- 1 cup water

  +
- ½ cup hibiscus water
- 1 cup cashews, soaked for 2 hours and rinsed
- ¼ cup Lakanto monk fruit sweetener, powdered
- 1 Tbsp orange juice
- ½ tsp sunflower lecithin
- 2 drops strawberry essence, alcohol-free
- 2 drops vanilla essence, alcohol-free
- 1 Tbsp agave nectar ➤

Hibiscus Filling Ingredients *(continued)*
- ½ tsp beet powder (for color)
- +
- ¼ cup coconut oil

Hibiscus Filling Instructions
1. Boil hibiscus flower with water for 2 minutes. Remove from stove and let cool down.
2. Blend all the second set of ingredients *(except coconut oil)* in blender.
3. Add coconut oil and blend again until a smooth consistency is obtained.
4. Remove cheesecake crust from freezer.
5. Pour equal amount of hibiscus filling into each of the two 4-inch springform pans.
6. Tap on counter to remove any air bubbles.
7. Place back in freezer overnight.

STRAWBERRY MACARONS

Macaron Crust Ingredients
- ½ cup of coconut flour (obtained by blending shredded coconut medium flakes into a powder form)
- ½ cup shredded coconut, medium flakes
- 1 Tbsp agave nectar or coconut nectar
- 1 pinch salt
- 5 drops vanilla extract, alcohol-free
- 2 drops strawberry extract, alcohol-free

Macaron Crust Instructions
1. Process crust ingredients in food processor until the batter starts sticking together.
2. Form small round balls with your hands, or use a round shaped cookie cutter. This will yield about 6-8 little round macarons.

3. Place on a lined dehydrator tray and dehydrate for 5 to 8 hours. Check periodically because the macaron should be slightly dry on the outside but soft on the inside.
4. When macarons are ready (dried on the outside but soft on the inside), put in refrigerator while making the macaron filling.

Filling Ingredients
- 1 cup strawberries, thawed
- 2 Tbsp agave nectar
- 1 pinch Himalayan sea salt

Filling Instructions
1. Add filling ingredients to a bowl.
2. Using a whisk, bring the ingredients to a chunky texture.
3. Dehydrate for 3 to 5 hours to make the jam more consistent.
4. Take 1 macaron crust, add about 1 tablespoon of macaron filling in center and cover with another macaron.
5. Put aside while making the pink glaze.

Pink Glaze Ingredients
- ¼ cup macadamia nuts, rinsed
- ½ cup cashews, soaked
- ½ cup almond milk
- 1 Tbsp monk fruit sweetener, powdered
- 2 Tbsp orange juice
- 1–2 tsp beet powder
- 5 drops strawberry extract
- 5 drops vanilla extract, alcohol-free
- ⅛ tsp Himalayan sea salt

+
- 1 Tbsp cacao butter, melted

Pink Glaze Instructions

1. Before you begin, bring Lakanto to powder in high-speed blender and set aside.
2. Add all the Pink Glaze ingredients to blender and blend until smooth.
3. Add melted cacao butter and blend again for a few seconds. Transfer glaze to glass bowl for dipping the macarons.
4. Cover each macaron (top and bottom) with the pink glaze mixture.
5. Place on a dehydrator sheet lined with parchment paper .
6. Place in refrigerator to firm up while making the vanilla frosting.

Vanilla Frosting Ingredients

- 1 cup cashews, soaked and rinsed
- ¼ cup almond water
- ¼ cup Lakanto monk fruit sweetener, powdered
- ½ Tbsp mesquite powder
- 1 Tbsp orange juice
- ¼ tsp orange zest
- 5 drops vanilla essence, alcohol-free
  +
- ¼ cup melted coconut oil

Vanilla Frosting Instructions

1. Blend all frosting ingredients (*except coconut oil*) until smooth.
2. Add coconut oil and blend again until well combined.
3. Allow to set in refrigerator for 12 to 24 hours before using.

ASSEMBLY

1. Remove hibiscus cheesecake from freezer.
2. Using a piping bag and a piping tip of your choice (1M *for example*), pipe a little bit of vanilla frosting on the cheesecake.
3. Top with a macaron.
4. Decorate with a candied citrus slice, pine berries or use an edible decoration of your choice.

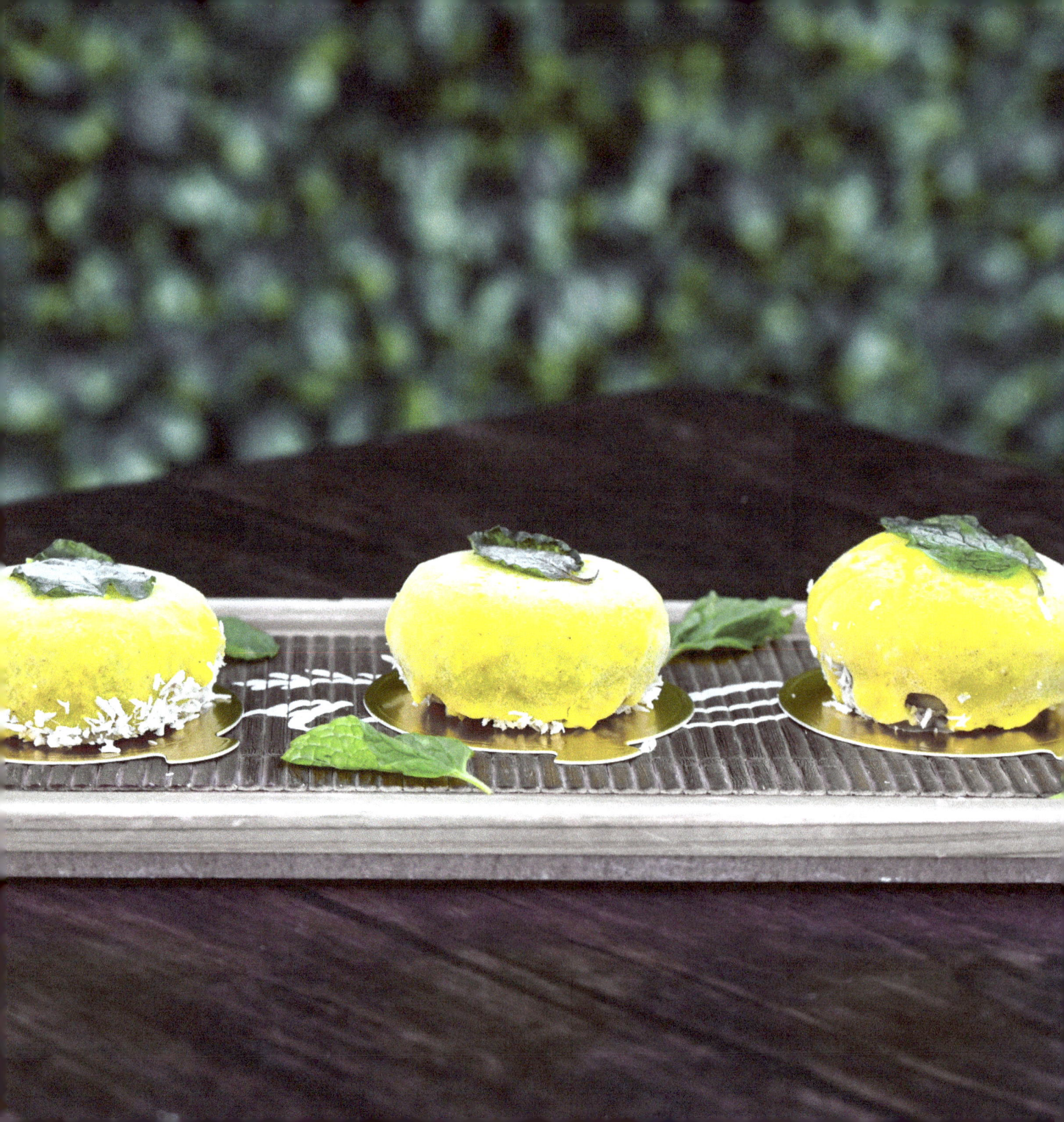

Tropical Pineapple Entremet

Serving size: 6 little round cakes

Equipment
- Food processor
- High-speed blender
- Stove
- Half sphere silicone mold
- Spoon
- Non-stick silicone mousse cake mold:
  11.7 inches long x 6.8 inches wide x 1.6 inches high
  (mold has 8 holes and has
  3D Stone round shape)
- Glass bowl
- Oven rack

Biscuit Ingredients
- 1 cup walnuts, soaked for 4 hours and dehydrated
- ½ cup dates, pitted
- ¼ cup coconut flakes (or medium shredded coconut)
- 3 drops vanilla extract
- ½ tsp orange, grated

Biscuit Instructions
1. Process ingredients until batter starts sticking together.
2. Set aside while making the jelly cake.

Pineapple Jelly Ingredients
- 1 cup pineapple, thawed
- ¼ Tbsp mineral salt
- ½ cup water
- 1 Tbsp coconut nectar
  +
- 2 Tbsp agar mixture
- 1 cup water

Pineapple Jelly Instructions
1. Blend first set of ingredients in high-speed blender until smooth. Pour into a glass bowl.
2. Bring second set of ingredients to a boil. Remove from stove. Let it cool down for a few minutes (do not wait until it gets hard) and add 2 tablespoons to first set of ingredients.
3. Pour into a half sphere silicone mold.
4. Place in freezer for at least 2 hours.

Brazil Nut Filling Ingredients
- ⅔ cup raw cashews, soaked for 2 hours and rinsed
- ¼ cup Brazil nuts, rinsed
- ½ cup almond milk
- 1 Tbsp mesquite powder
- 1 peach, de-seeded
- 1 Tbsp orange juice ➤

Brazil Nut Filling Instructions

1. Blend all ingredients until smooth.
2. Remove pineapple jelly from molds.
3. Using a spoon, pour Brazil nut filling into each cavity of Non-stick silicone mousse cake mold up to ⅓ of the mold.
4. Add pineapple jelly into each mold. Then, cover up with Brazil nut filling again, leaving 1 each out for the biscuit base.
5. Add the biscuit crumble on top of the Brazil nut filling for each cavity. Leave the remainder for the strawberry raw cake.
6. Tap on the counter to remove air bubbles. Freeze for 5 hours minimum or overnight.

Turmeric Chocolate Enrobing Ingredients

- ½ cup Brazil nuts, rinsed
- ¼ cup almond milk at room temperature
- 1 Tbsp Lakanto, powdered or monk fruit sweetener
- 1 Tbsp orange juice
- 5 drops vanilla essence, alcohol-free
- 1 tsp turmeric powder
- 1 Tbsp coconut nectar
  +
- ⅓ cup melted coconut butter

Turmeric Chocolate Enrobing Instructions

1. Blend all ingredients (*except the butter*) in high-speed blender until smooth.
2. Add melted coconut butter and blend again until smooth.
3. Pour into a bowl for dripping.
4. Remove entremet from freezer.
5. Put glass bowl underneath an oven rack.
6. Put entremet (one at a time) on top of rack.
7. Slowly pour the turmeric chocolate enrobing mixture on top until fully covered.
8. Repeat the operation until all entremets are covered with mixture.
9. Place back in refrigerator for 1 hour to set. Remove and enjoy.
10. Store in freezer for up to 1 month.

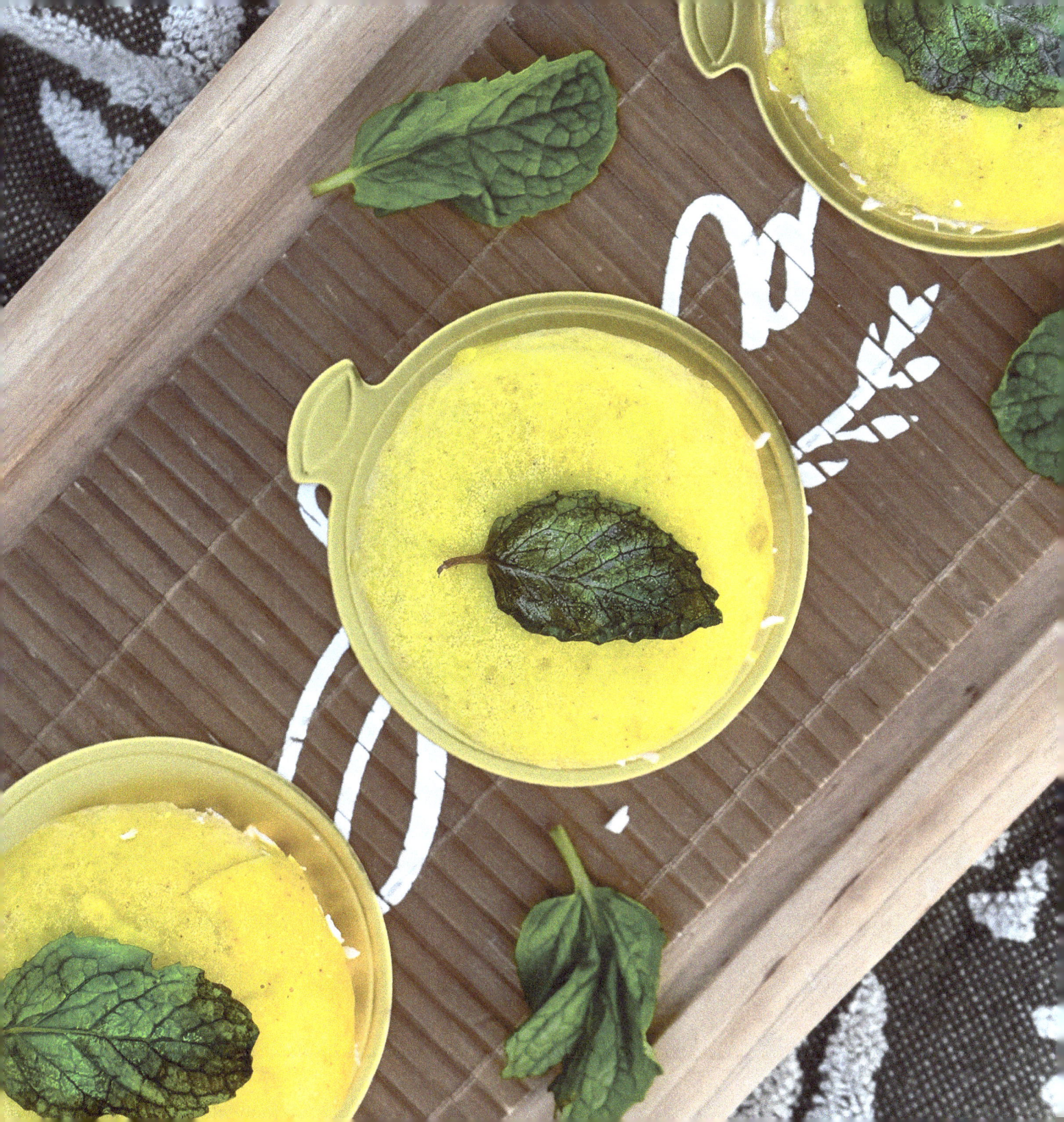

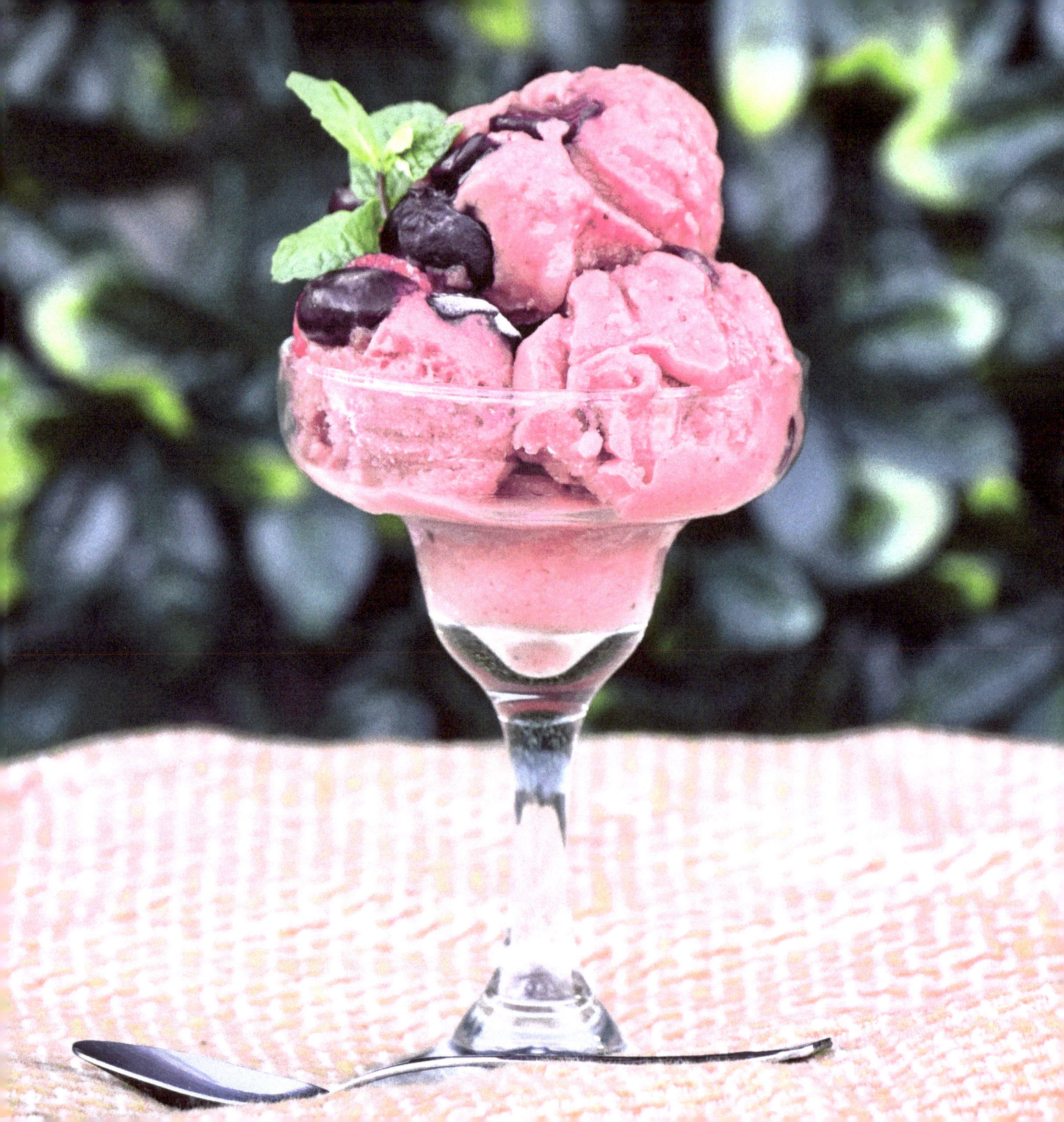

Strawberry Frozen Ice Cream

Serving size: 1

Equipment

- Bowl
- High-speed blender
- Bowl
- Cup
- Ice cream scoop
- Ice cream Ingredients
- ½ cup organic mangoes, frozen
- 1 cup frozen organic strawberries (you can add more for more sweetness)
- ½ cup coconut milk
- 3 Tbsp coconut nectar

Topping Ingredients

1 cup organic cherries, fresh

Instructions

1. Blend first set of ingredients (without the cherries).
2. Add to a bowl. Use a scoop to scoop it out like ice cream balls and add to a cup.
3. Add cherries as topping. Serve immediately.
4. If the mixture is too liquid, put in freezer for 1 hour, then remove from freezer before you scoop it out.

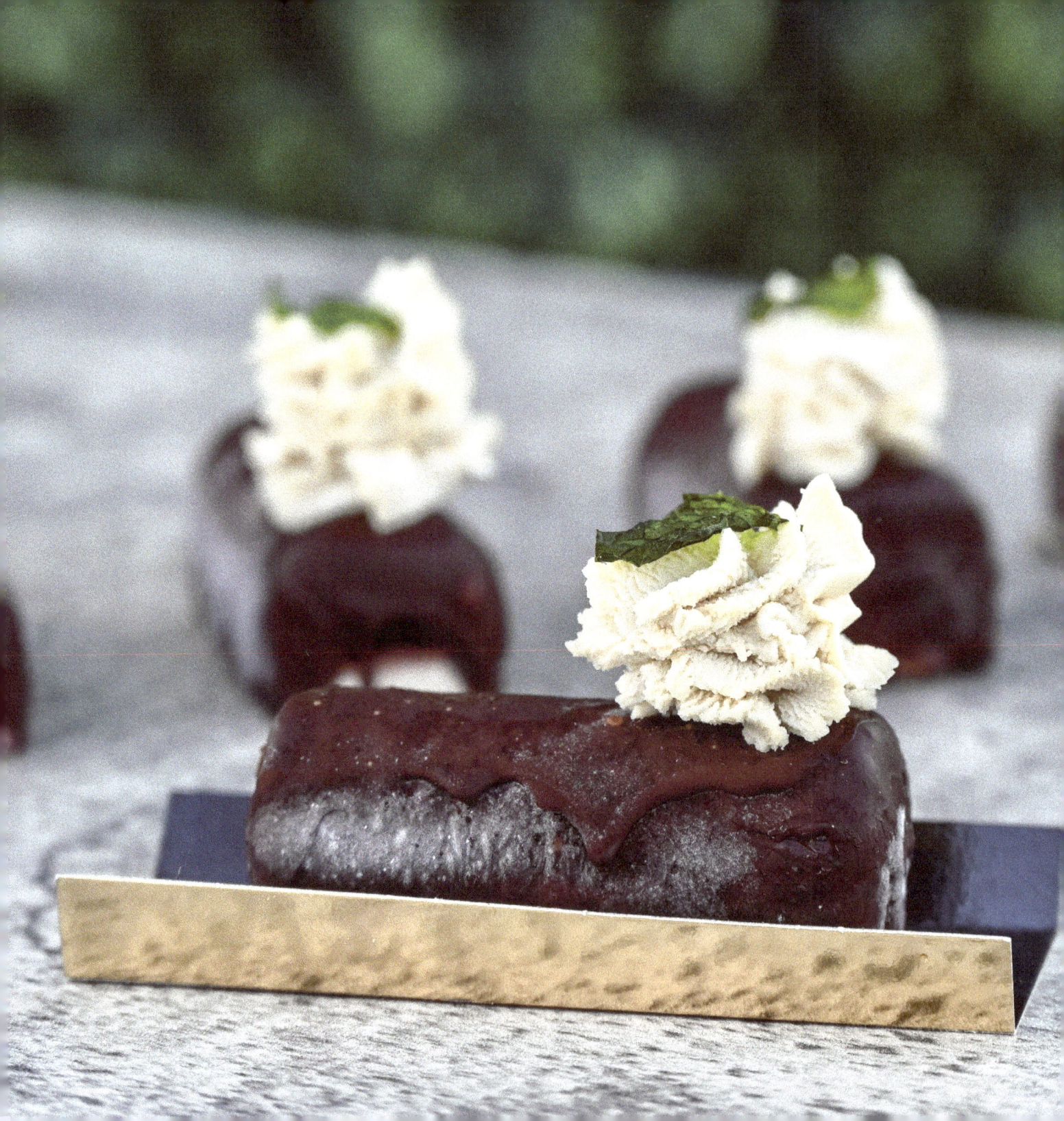

Raw Coconut Bar

Serving size: 7–9 bars

Equipment

- Food processor
- 9-cavities log mold (each log mold measures approximately 3.31 inches long, 1.26 inches wide, and 1.38 inches high)
- Shallow container
- Whisk
- Stove
- Double boiler pot
- Food grade gloves
- Toothpick

Crumble Ingredients

- 1 cup walnuts, soaked for 4 hours and dehydrated
- 1 cup desiccated shredded coconut
- ¼ cup dates, soaked
- ¼ cup dates, pitted and soaked
  +
- 2 Tbsp coconut oil, melted

Crumble Instructions

1. Process ingredients (except the coconut oil) in food processor until batter starts sticking together.
2. Add the coconut oil and process again.
3. Add to the bottom of the silicone mold. Set aside.

Raspberry Filling Ingredients

- 1 cup raspberries, fresh
- 2 Tbsp maple syrup or agave nectar
- 1 or 2 drops vanilla essence, alcohol-free

Raspberry Filling Instructions

1. Put ingredients into a shallow container. Using a whisk, bring them to a creamy texture.
2. Remove silicone mold from the freezer and add raspberry filling on top.
3. Place in freezer for a minimum of 6 hours.

Coconut Cream Ingredients

- 1 cup cashew nuts, soaked for 2 hours and rinsed
- ¼ cup agave nectar
- 2 Tbsp vanilla essence, alcohol-free
- ½ cup desiccated shredded coconut
- ½ cup almond milk (add an additional ¼ cup almond milk as needed)
- ¼ cup coconut butter, melted

Coconut Cream Instructions

1. Blend the coconut cream ingredients until smooth.
2. Add to the silicone mold and place in freezer while working on the next layer. ➤

Chocolate Shell Ingredients

- ½ cup cacao paste, melted (using the double boiler method)
- ¼ cup cacao butter
- 3 Tbsp agave nectar
- 1 or 2 drops vanilla essence, alcohol-free

Chocolate Shell Instructions

1. Melt cacao paste and butter using the double boiler.
2. When the coconut bar is firm enough, remove from freezer and unmold.
3. Put on the gloves for the enrobing process; otherwise the chocolate will melt quickly in your hands. Get a toothpick ready.
4. To enrobe the bars with chocolate, insert the toothpick in the middle of each bar and dip into the chocolate mixture. Do not dip the bottom of the bar.
5. Place on a lined tray. Repeat the operation until all bars are covered.
6. Return to the freezer for 15 minutes while making the vanilla cream frosting from the refrigerator for decoration of the bars.

Vanilla Cream Frosting Ingredients

- 1 cup cashews, soaked for 2 hours and rinsed (*or substitute walnuts*)
- ¼ cup coconut milk
- ¼ cup coconut nectar
- 1 Tbsp orange juice or any citrus juice
- 5 drops vanilla essence, alcohol-free
- ½ cup coconut oil or cacao butter, melted
- 1 bouquet mint leaf for decoration

Vanilla Cream Frosting Instructions

1. Blend vanilla cream frosting ingredients (*except coconut oil*) in high-speed blender until smooth.
2. Add coconut oil and blend again.
3. Pour into a shallow container.
4. Refrigerate for 12 to 24 hours.
5. Using a piping bag with a Milton 1B piping tip, decorate coconut bar and add a leaf mint on top of each dollop as per the picture.
6. Enjoy immediately or put in the freezer for up to 1 month.

Notes: _____

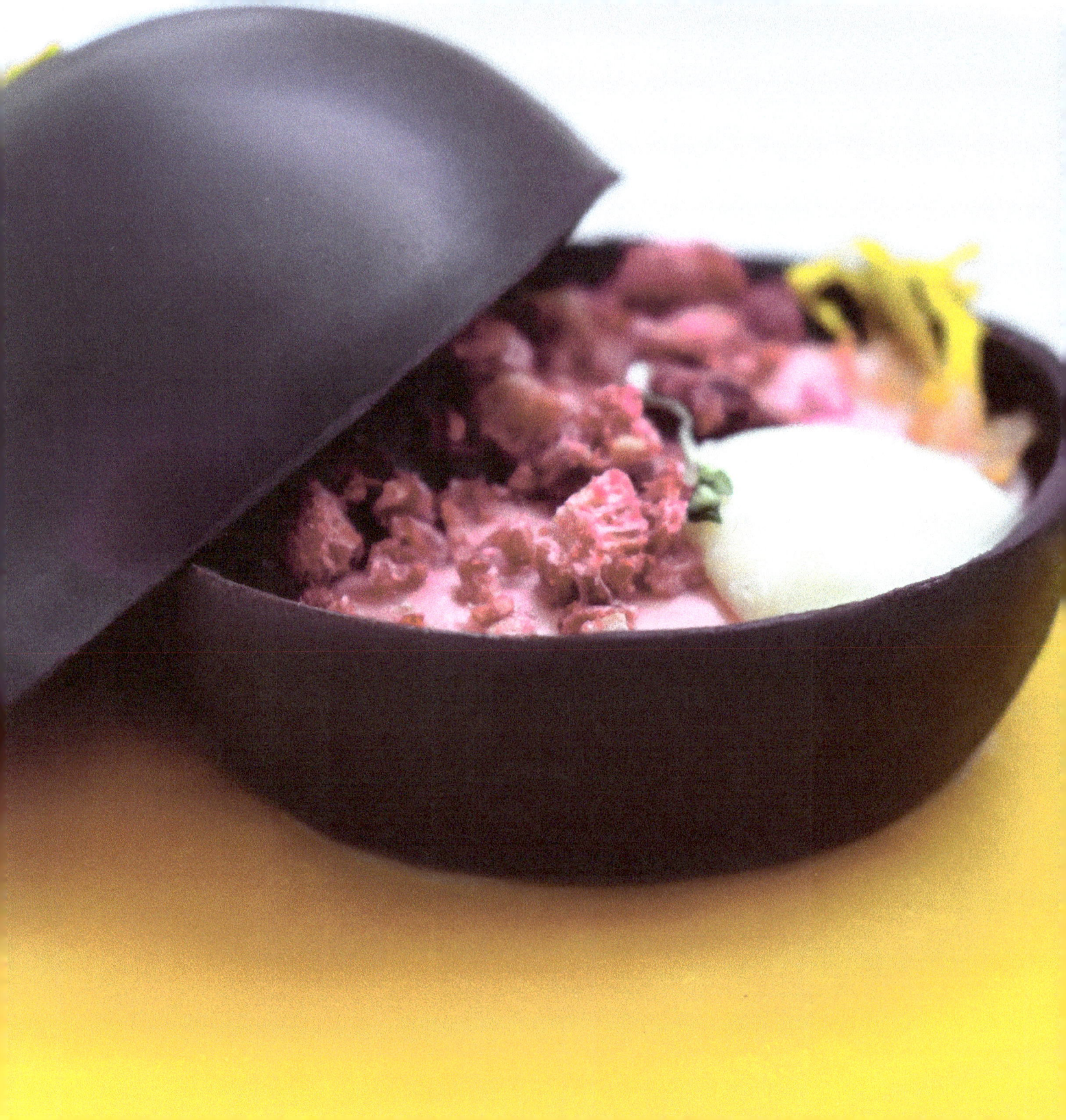

X
BONUS RECIPES
RAW DESSERTS

Taking your raw dessert skills to the next level!

Making creative raw desserts can be a healing experience for some and a challenge for others. Whatever that represents to you, it is always rewarding to learn how to make your own food and attempt to create unique recipes you will share with your loved ones.

Eating raw food helps in gaining more energy since vitamins and minerals contained in the foods are not destroyed by the cooking process.

Raw desserts are easy to digest since they are gluten-free, egg-free and dairy-free. Each ingredient has been intentionally used for its nutritional value and taste.

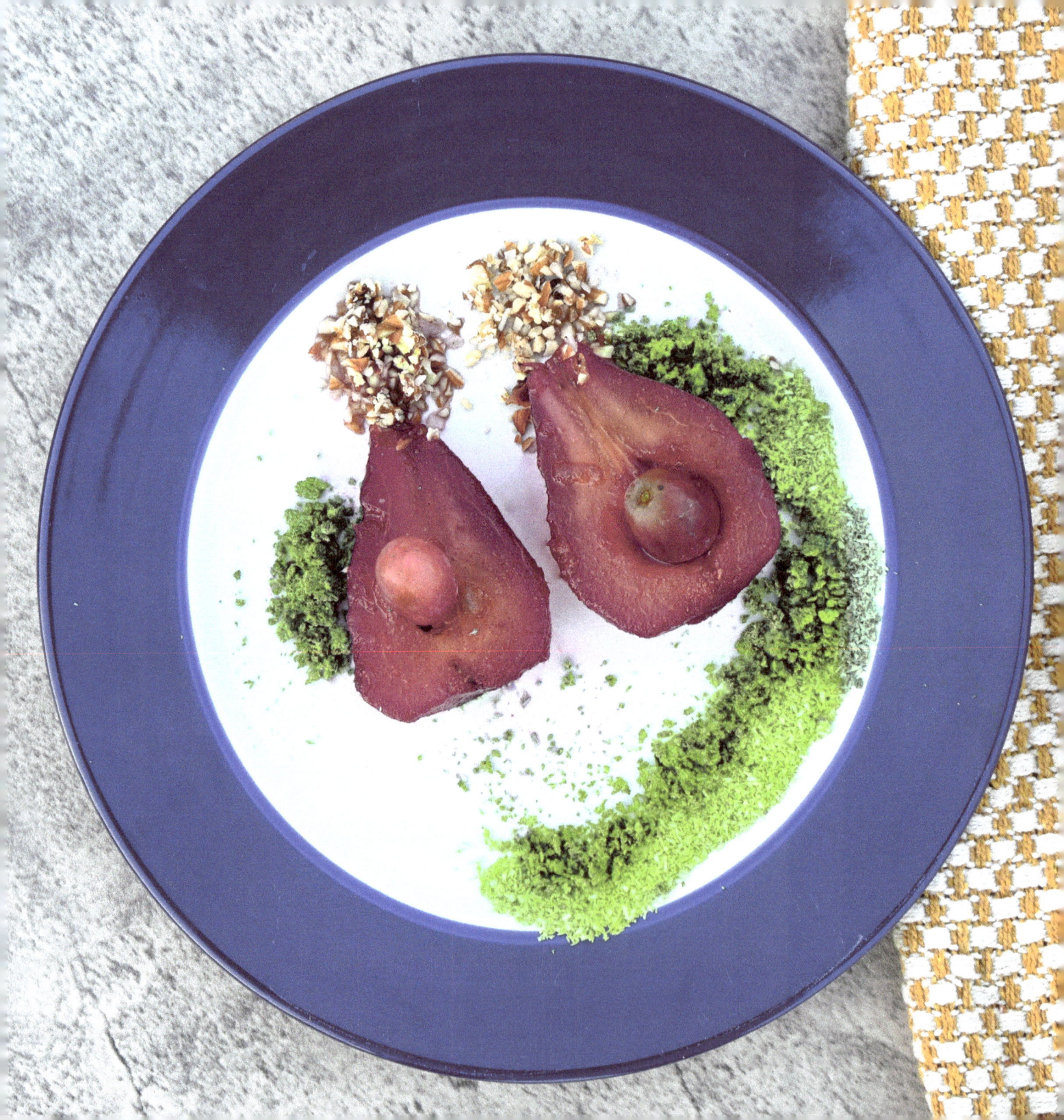

Hibiscus Poached Pear

Serving size: 1

Equipment

- Cooking pan
- Stove
- High-speed blender
- Glass mixing bowl
- Dehydrator
- Parchment paper
- Knife

Candied Coconut Sprinkles Ingredients

- 3 cups coconut, shredded (1 cup for each color)
- ¼ cup cane sugar, powdered
- 1 tsp turmeric powder
  +
- 3 cups coconut, shredded (1 cup for each color)
- ¼ cup cane sugar, powdered
- 1 tsp matcha powder

Candied Coconut Sprinkles Instructions

1. Soak coconut in enough water to cover it for 4 hours until softened.
2. Strain with fine-mesh strainer.
3. Add powdered cane sugar and divide into 3 equal parts.

4. For the yellow color, add 1 cup coconut to the mixing bowl and mix well with the turmeric powder.
5. Add to a dehydrator lined with parchment paper and dehydrate for 8 hours at 115°F (46°C).
6. Repeat the same process for the matcha powder and beet powder.

Candied Nuts Ingredients

- 2 cups of nuts of your choice (almonds or cashews), soaked and dehydrated
- ¾ cup powdered coconut sugar (powdered in a blender)
- 1 Tbsp orange juice
- 12 drops vanilla essence, alcohol-free
- ⅛ tsp high mineral salt

Candied Nuts Instructions

1. Soak nuts for 2 to 4 hours and strain them.
2. Add all ingredients to a food processor and pulse for few seconds until chunky. Add to mixing bowl and mix until well combined.
3. Place on a parchment paper-lined dehydrator and dehydrate for 24 to 36 hours at 115°F (46°C). ➤

Poached Pear Ingredients

- 1 cup water, room temperature
- ¼ cup hibiscus flower

  +
- ¼ cup of organic cane sugar
- 1 Tbsp mesquite powder (optional)
- 1 Tbsp organic beet powder (for a stronger red color)
- 5 tsp vanilla extract (non-alcohol brand)

  +
- 1 ripe organic pear

  +
- 2 individual grapes (purple color)

Poached Pear Instructions

1. Pour water and hibiscus flower into cooking pan and bring to boil for 5 minutes, until color of the water starts changing.
2. Remove from stove and let cool.
3. Add remaining ingredients (*except the pear and grapes*) to hibiscus water and mix together until combined.
4. Peel the pear. Cut it in half and remove the seeds.
5. Pour hibiscus water into a glass mixing bowl and add the 2 halves of pear to it.
6. Refrigerate for at least 4 to 5 hours. This process helps the pears to soften by absorbing the hibiscus water.
7. Remove pears from refrigerator and take them out of the hibiscus water. Set aside.

ASSEMBLY

1. Add the 2 pear halves to a plate (*see picture on previous page*).
2. Take ¼ of candied matcha coconut sprinkles and create an arch around the poached pears. You can use a mix of colors for the decoration as needed. Put the remainder in a sealed bag and store in freezer for future use.
3. Add the thinly sliced pears next to the 2 halves.
4. Add 1 tablespoon of candied nuts at the top of each half pear and add 1 grape in the center of each of them.
5. Serve right away.
6. Storage: Store in refrigerator for up to 3 days only due to the freshness of the fruits.

Notes: _____

_____

_____

_____

_____

_____

_____

_____

_____

_____

_____

_____

_____

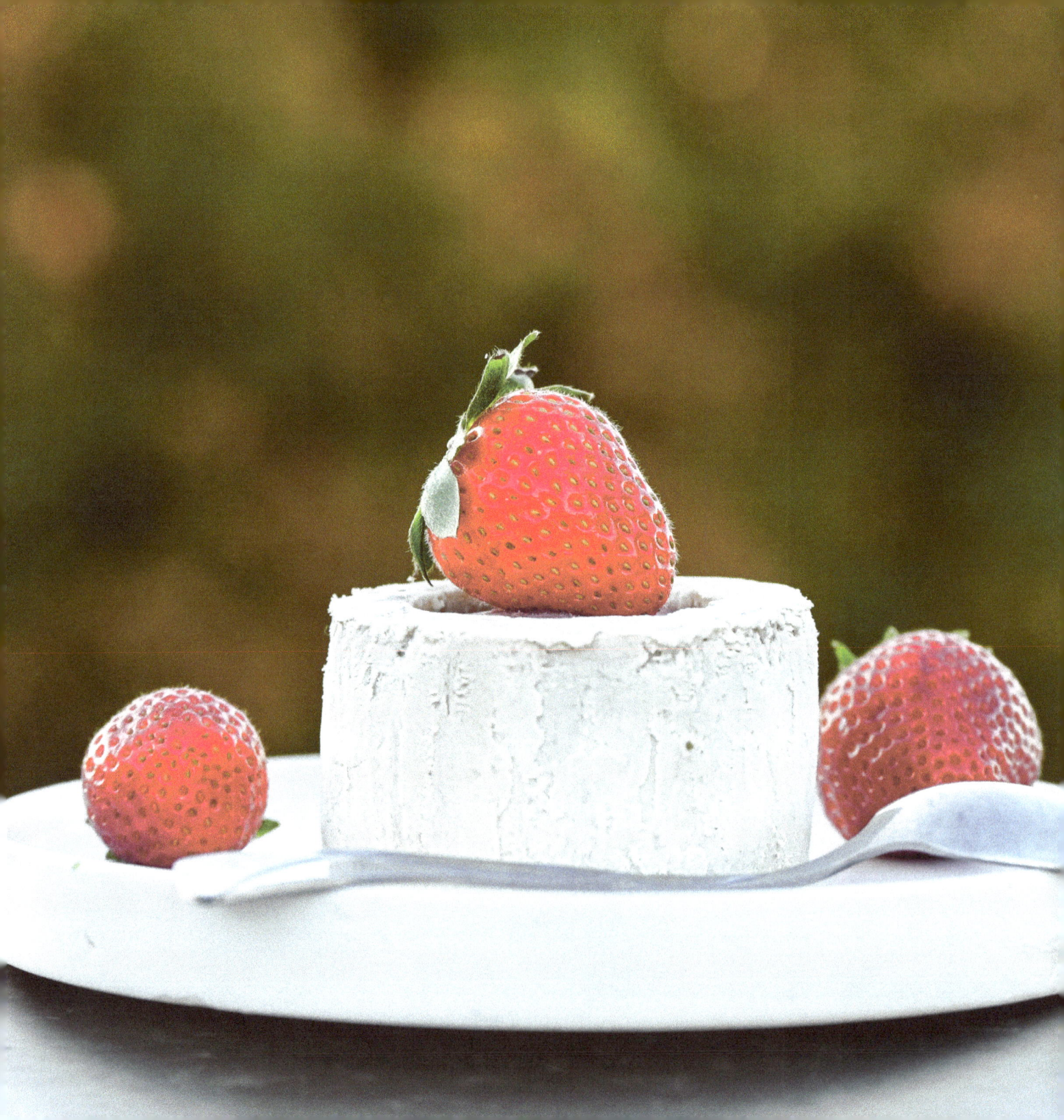

Strawberry Raw Cake

Serving size: 4 (small cakes)

Equipment

- High-speed blender
- Truffle Pudding bomb silicone mold
  (1) 11.7 inches x 6.8 inches x 1.6 inches
- Food processor
- Mixing bowl
- Knife

Crumble Cake (*base*)

Use remaining from the "Tropical Pineapple Entremet"

Orange Cheesecake Filling Ingredients

- 1 cup cashews
- ¼ cup coconut flakes or shredded coconut
- ½ cup dates
- ½ cup to 1 cup water (as needed to blend)
- 5 drops vanilla essence, alcohol-free
- •¼ tsp orange, grated
- ⅛ tsp pinch of salt
  +
- 1 Tbsp coconut oil, melted

Orange Cheesecake Filling Instructions

1. Blend Orange Cheesecake ingredients (*except coconut oil*).
2. Add coconut oil and blend again until smooth.
3. Pour orange filling into large round part of the mold.
4. Tap gently on the counter (to remove air bubbles)
5. Place in freezer for 5 hours or overnight.

6. **Strawberry Filling Ingredients**

- 1 cup cashews, soaked for 2 hours and rinsed
- 1 cup whole strawberries, fresh
- ½ cup pitted dates
- ½ cup water (as needed to blend)
- 5 drops vanilla essence
- juice of 1 whole orange
- ⅛ tsp salt
- 1 tsp beetroot powder
  +
- 1 Tbsp coconut oil, melted
  +
- 4 strawberries for decoration ➤

Strawberry Filling Instructions

1. Add the Strawberry Filling ingredients (*except the melted coconut oil*) to a high-speed blender and blend until smooth.
2. Add the coconut oil and blend again.
3. Remove cake from freezer.
4. Pour the strawberry layer on the opposite part of the mold (small round part of mold)
5. Put back in freezer for a minimum of 2 hours.

ASSEMBLY

1. Remove from freezer.
2. Press Crumble Cake Base mixture gently into top of the cake mold (large round part).
3. Put back in freezer for 1 hour to firm up.
4. Remove from freezer and remove cakes from molds.
5. Let thaw for a few minutes
6. Add one strawberry on top of strawberry filling.
7. Serve and enjoy or store in freezer for up to 1 month.

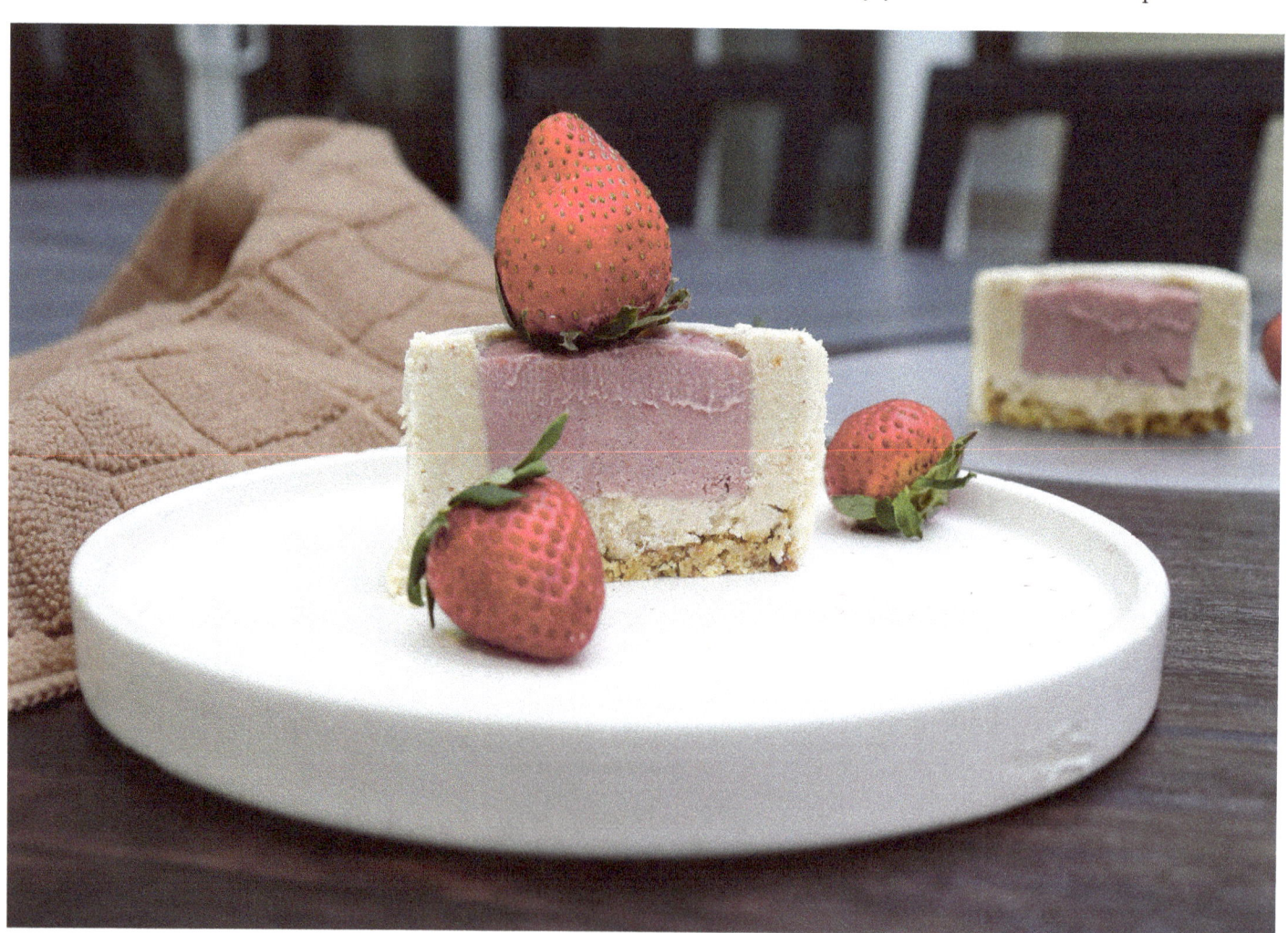

Notes: _____

_____

_____

_____

_____

_____

_____

_____

_____

_____

_____

_____

_____

_____

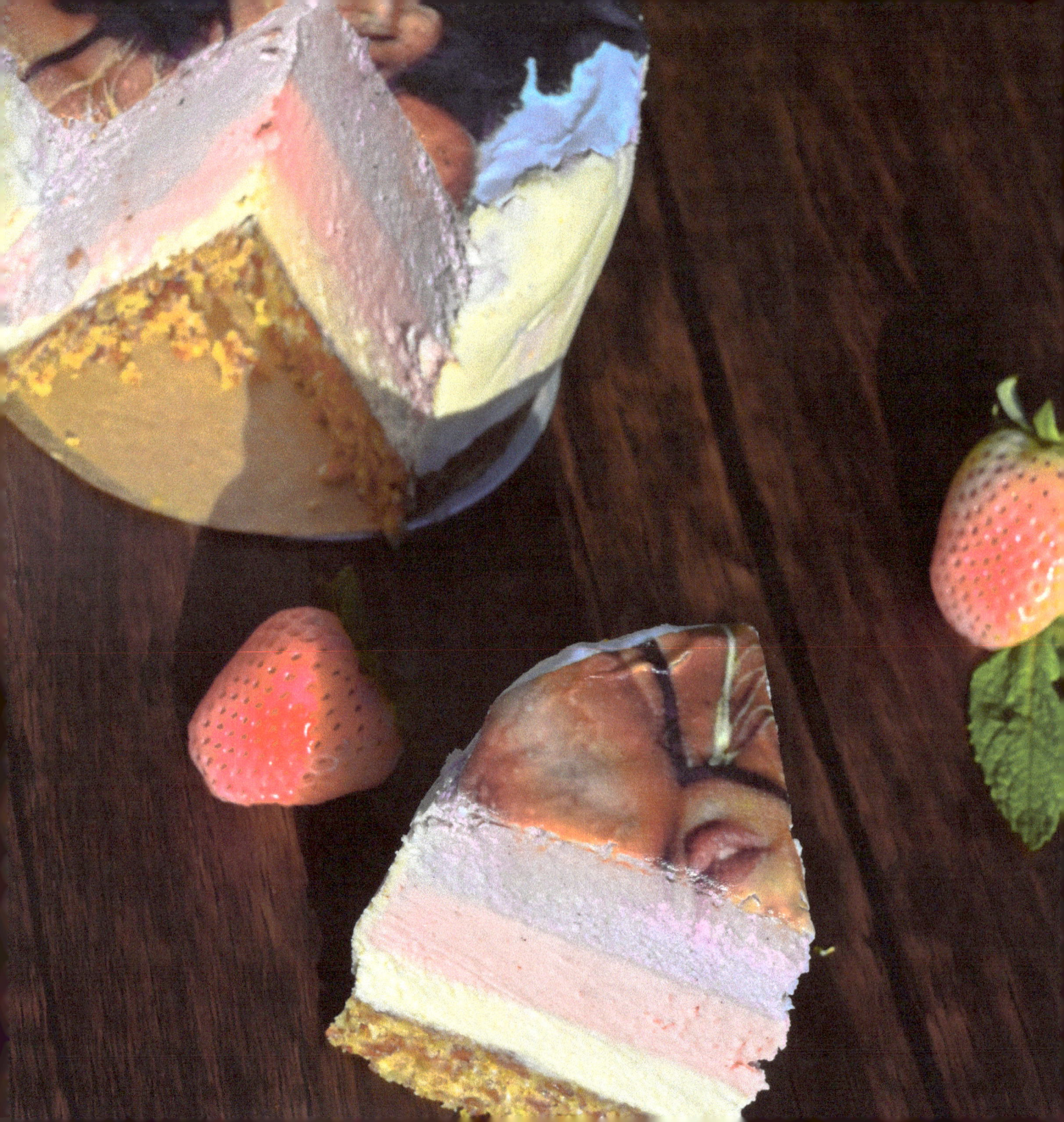

Strawberry Hibiscus Cheesecake

Serving size:1

Equipment

- High-speed blender
- Food processor
- 6-inch springform pan
- Cake turntable
- 4-inch clear cake acetate roll or acetate strips
- Tape
- Spatula
- Scraper
- Cake turntable
- Stove
- Pan
- Shallow container
- Edible dairy-free and gluten-free cake topper

Walnut Crust Ingredients

- 1 cup walnuts, soaked for 4 hours, rinsed and dehydrated
- 1 cup Medjool dates
- ¼ cup coconut, shredded
- 1 Tbsp orange juice
- 3 drops vanilla extract
- Pinch of salt

Walnut Crust Instructions

1. Using the acetate roll, form a round shape to measure how much will be needed to cover the inside of the mold.
2. Remove and cut with scissors.
3. Repeat the process again.
4. Place one acetate strip on top of the other and secure them with a tape. This is necessary because the cake will be tall so we want to prevent any spill.
5. Use the acetate strips to line the inside of the cake mold.
6. Process ingredients in food processor until batter starts sticking together.
7. Pour into 6-inch springform pan and place in freezer while making the filling.

Vanilla Cream Filling Ingredients

- 1 cup cashews, soaked for 2 hours and rinsed
- ¼ cup coconut milk
- 3 Tbsp agave nectar
- ¼ cup orange juice
- 4 drops vanilla essence
  +
- ⅛ cup coconut oil, melted ➤

Vanilla Cream Filling Instructions

1. Blend all ingredients (*except the coconut oil*) in a blender until smooth.
2. Add coconut oil and blend again for smoother consistency.
3. Remove the springform pan from freezer
4. Pour vanilla cream on top of the crust.
5. Tap on the counter to remove air bubbles
6. Place back into freezer for at least 1 hour while making the strawberry filling.

Strawberry Filling Ingredients

- 1 cup cashews, soaked for 2 hours and rinsed
- ¼ cup coconut milk
- ¼ cup organic agave nectar or coconut nectar
- ¼ cup orange juice
- ½ tsp organic beet powder
- 4 drops vanilla essence, alcohol-free
- 3 drops strawberry essence, alcohol-free
  +
- ¼ cup coconut oil, melted

Strawberry Filling Instructions

1. Blend all ingredients (except the coconut oil) in a blender until smooth.
2. Add the coconut oil and blend again for a smoother consistency.
3. Remove the springform pan from the freezer and pour strawberry filling on top of vanilla cream layer.
4. Tap on the counter to remove any air bubbles and place back into freezer for at least 1 hour while making the hibiscus filling.

Hibiscus Filling Ingredients

- 1 cup cashews, soaked for 2 hours and rinsed
- ¼ cup almond milk
- ¼ cup agave nectar
- ¼ cup orange juice
- 2 Tbsp hibiscus tea(obtained by boiling 1 cup of water with
  ¼ cup of hibiscus flower and cooling down.
  You will only need 2 Tbsp.
  Store the remaining in refrigerator)
- 1 tsp Maqui berry powder (*optional for the extra purple color*)
- 4 drops vanilla essence, alcohol-free
- ¼ cup coconut oil, melted

Hibiscus Filling Instructions

1. Blend all ingredients (*except the coconut oil*) in a blender until smooth.
2. Add the coconut oil and blend again for a smoother consistency.
3. Remove the springform pan from the freezer.
4. Pour hibiscus filling on the strawberry cream layer.
5. Tap on the counter to remove any air bubbles.
6. Place back into the freezer for 6 hours or overnight.

Vanilla Frosting Ingredients

- 1 cup cashews, soaked for 2 hours and rinsed
- ¼ cup coconut milk
- ¼ cup agave nectar
- 2 tsp orange juice
- 1 tsp orange zest
- 4 drops vanilla essence, alcohol-free
  +
- ¼ cup coconut oil, melted

Vanilla Frosting Instructions

1. Blend all ingredients (except the coconut oil) in a blender until smooth.
2. Add coconut oil and blend again for a smoother consistency.
3. Pour into a shallow container and place in the refrigerator to set for 12 to 24 hours.

ASSEMBLY

1. Remove cake from freezer and from springform pan.
2. Remove acetate strips too.
3. Remove vanilla frosting from the freezer.
4. Frost the cake on a cake turntable using the vanilla frosting.
5. Place the cake back in the freezer overnight.

DECORATION

1. Remove cake from the freezer.
2. Add an edible African decoration sheet *(may be ordered online)* or any edible decoration of your choice on top of the cake.
3. Serve immediately or store in refrigerator for up to 1 week or in freezer for up to 1 month.
4. *Note: The edible African decoration might not last more than a couple days in the refrigerator or freezer but the cake itself will.*

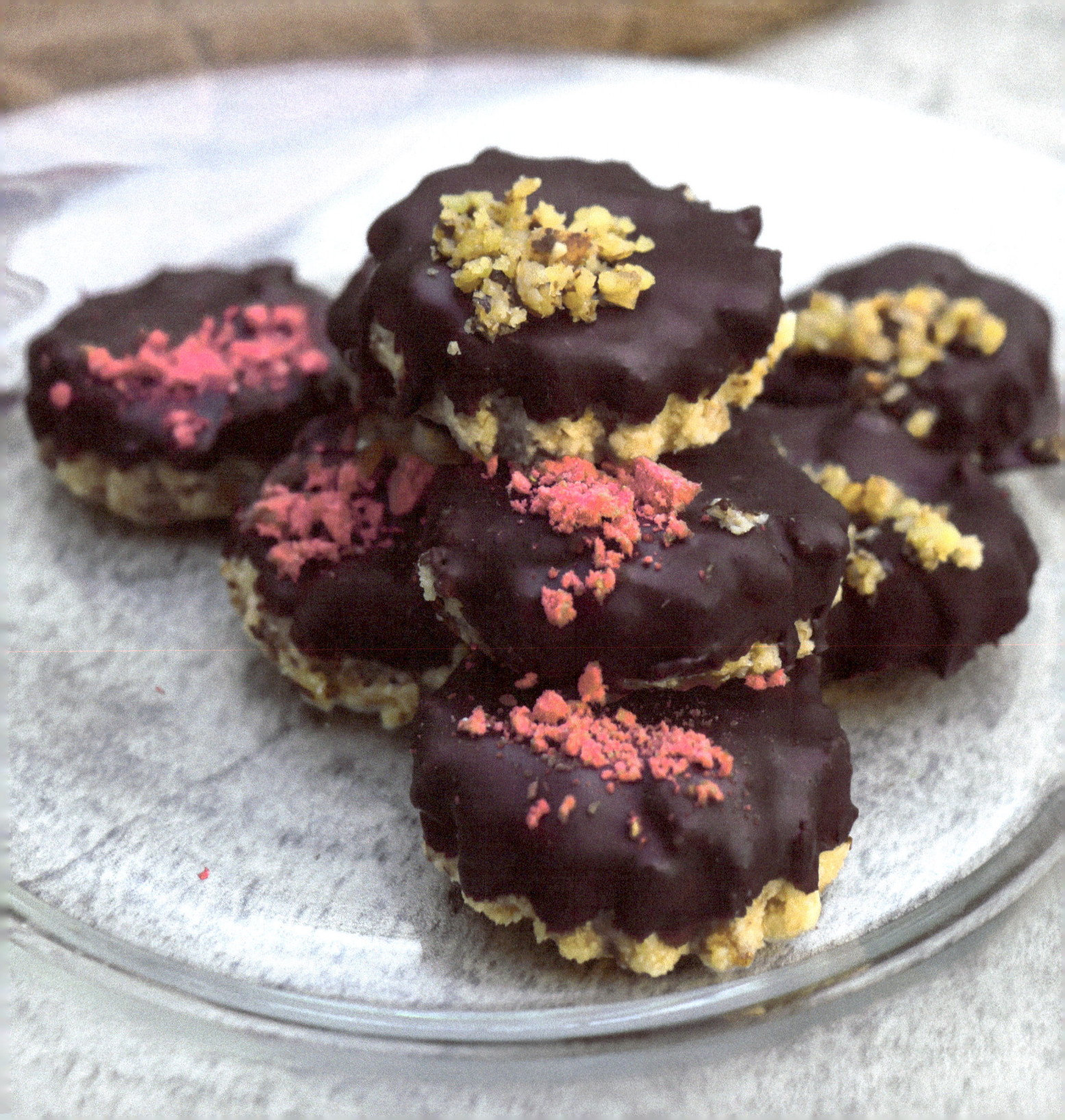

Raw Almond Cookies

Serving size: 13 little cookies

Equipment

- Spatula
- Glass bowl
- Double boiler pot
- Cutting board
- Cookie cutter (round shape)
- Fork
- Parchment paper

Cookie Crust Ingredients

- 2 cups almond pulp, wet
- ¼ cup shredded coconut
- ¼ cup agave nectar, raw
- 1 Tbsp mesquite powder
- 1 Tbsp clementine juice
- 3 drops vanilla essence, alcohol-free
- ⅛ tsp of Himalayan sea salt

Cookie Crust Instructions

1. Mix all ingredients in a bowl using a spatula.
2. Using a cookie cutter, make round shaped cookies.
3. Put in freezer for at least 45 minutes while making the glaze.

Glaze Ingredients

- ⅔ cup shaved cacao paste
- ⅓ cup shaved cacao butter
- 6 Tbsp coconut nectar
- 5 drops vanilla extract, alcohol-free
- ⅛ tsp of Himalayan sea salt

    +
- ¼ cup citrus crumble (from the Raw Mango Crumble recipe, *next page*) or powdered, freeze-dried strawberries

Glaze Instructions

1. Melt cacao paste and butter using double boiler method.
2. Remove mixture from stove.
3. Add coconut nectar, vanilla extract and sea salt. Mix together with a spatula.
4. Let cool for 30 minutes before enrobing. We want to avoid enrobing the cookies with hot chocolate.

ASSEMBLY

1. Remove cookies from freezer
2. Using a fork, enrobe only one side of each cookie.
3. Put on a cutting board lined with parchment paper
4. Using your hands, sprinkle quickly with a tsp of remaining citrus crumble or with powdered freeze dried strawberries.
5. Put back in freezer for 30 minutes to firm up.
6. Remove from freezer when ready to enjoy.
7. Store in freezer for up to 1 month.

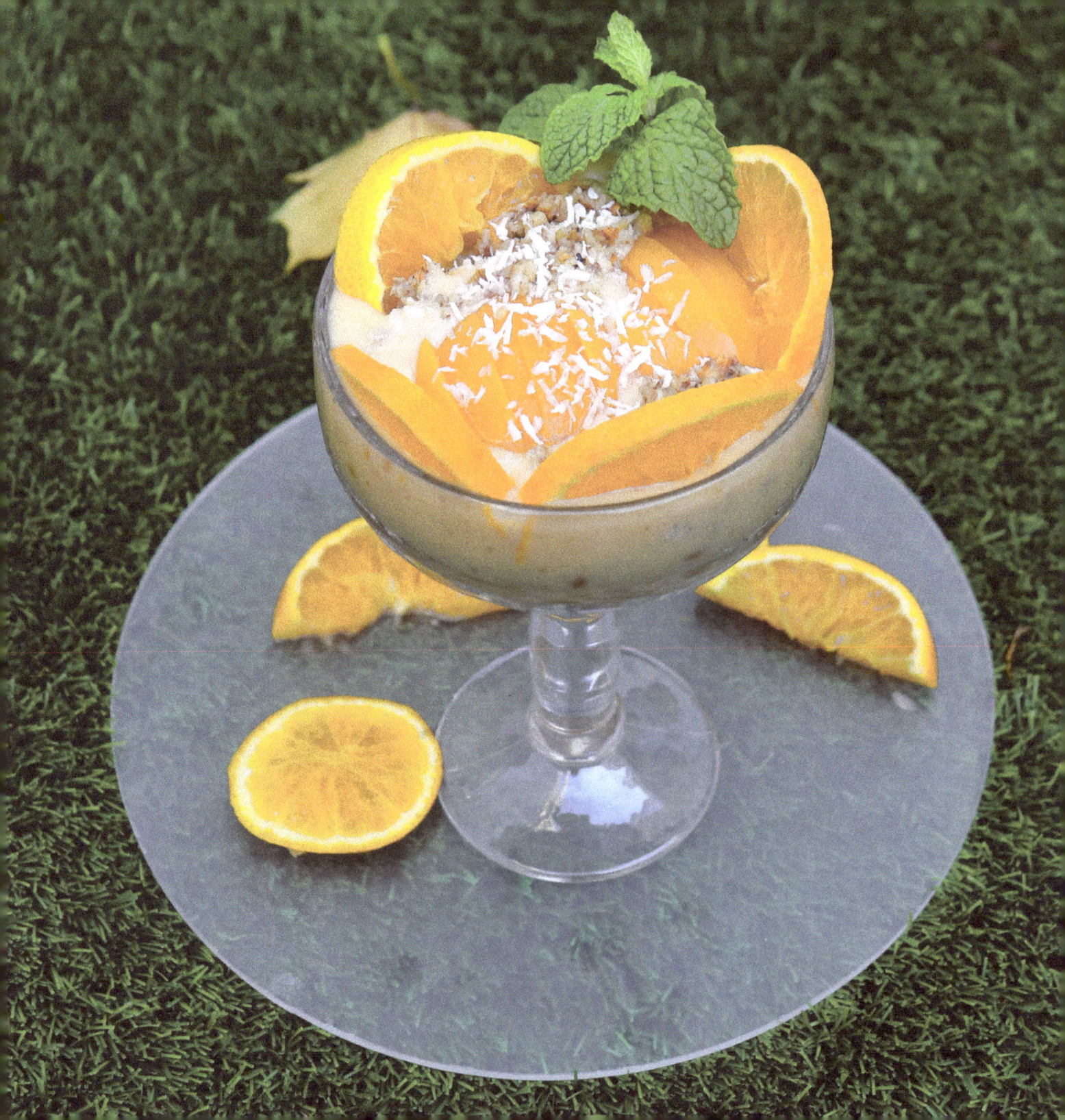

Raw Mango Crumble

Serving size:1

Equipment
- Food processor
- High-speed blender
- Glass bowl

Citrus Crumble Ingredients
- ¼ cup almonds
- ⅔ cup walnuts
- 1 Tbsp mesquite powder
- 1 Tbsp juice of a clementine
- ⅛ tsp Himalayan sea salt
- 5 drops non-alcoholic vanilla extract
  +
- 1 Tbsp cacao butter or coconut oil, melted
  +
- ¾ cup raw peaches, sliced to ¼ inch wide
- 2 Tbsp shredded coconut

Citrus Crumble Instructions
1. Process the first set of ingredients in food processor until you get a chunky texture.
2. Add cacao butter and process again for a few seconds. Do not overprocess as we still want to see the texture looking like a crumble.
3. Add to a mixing bowl and set aside.

Mango Smoothie Ingredients
- 1 cup mangoes, frozen
- ¾ cup coconut milk (obtain by blending 2 cups water and 1 cup desiccated coconut, then straining to separate the milk from the pulp)
- 3 organic dates, pitted

Mango Smoothie Instructions
1. Add frozen mangoes, coconut milk and dates to a high-speed blender and blend until smooth.
2. Add the mango smoothie mixture to a glass bowl until it is ¾ filled. ➤

ASSEMBLY

Assembly Ingredients

- ¼ cup of sliced peaches
- 1 orange

Assembly Instructions

1. Add about half of the crumble mixture in the middle of the bowl.
2. Add sliced peaches on top of crumble.
3. Add remaining crumble on top of sliced peaches.
4. Sprinkle with shredded coconut.
5. Decorate with oranges or any citrus of your choice, pre-cut into half spheres and thin slices.
6. Add each half of the thinly cut oranges to the edges of the smoothie bowl until you create a full circle of citrus orange around the bowl.
7. Refrigerate for 20 minutes before serving.
8. Store in refrigerator for up to 1 week.

Notes: _____

_____

_____

_____

_____

_____

_____

_____

_____

_____

_____

_____

_____

_____

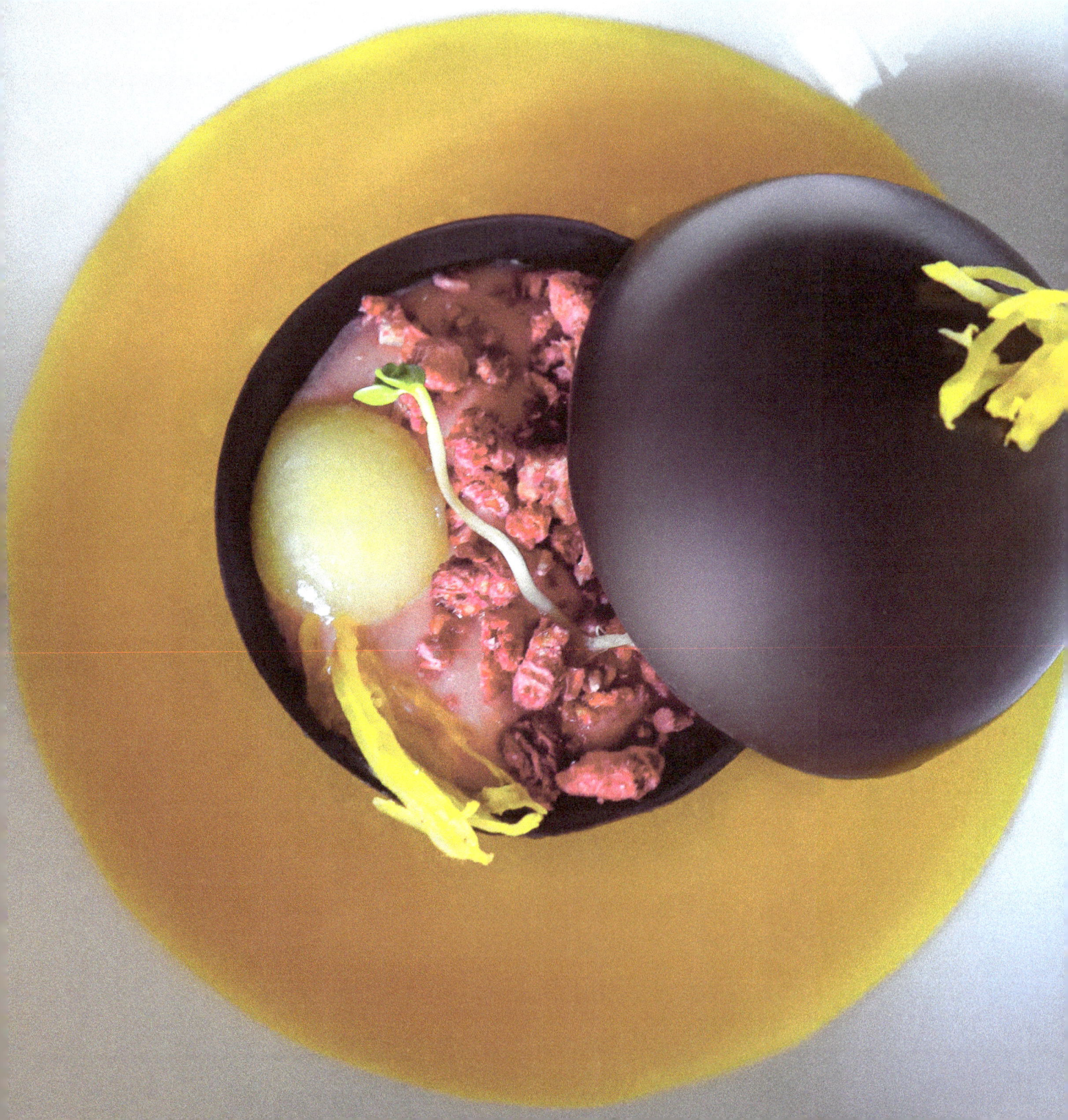

Pumpkin Latte Bomb

Serving size: 1
Yield: 6 half spheres including 1 full serving of pumpkin latte bomb.

The Ingredients are listed, not in order of importance, but in order of category for easy identification in each part of the recipe. It is important that you gather the right quantities. You can eventually alter some Ingredients, depending upon your taste, but the quantities should be similar.

Equipment

- A round silicone mold 11.6 x 6.9 x 1.3 inches
  (29.5 x 17.5 x 3.3 cm);
  hole diameter: 2.55 inches (6.5 cm)
- Small silicone mold 9 x 2.75 x 0.9 inches
- Double boiler pot
- Spatula
- A brownie silicone mold
  (1 pc: 24-Cavity: 8.5 x 13.2 x 0.6 inch)
- 3 shallow containers
- High-speed blender
- Pan (any size but recommended is 13.75 x 7.75 x
  7.25 inches)
- Chocolate brush
- Mixing bowl
- Digital thermometer
- Round shape white plate for presentation
- Tweezers
  The high-speed blender and the digital thermometer reader are essential to make this recipe a success

Little Chocolate Spheres Ingredients

- ½ cup cacao butter, melted
- ½ cup macadamia nuts, rinsed
- ⅓ cup coconut oil
- 3 Tbsp light agave nectar
- 5 drops vanilla essence, alcohol-free
- ⅛ tsp Himalayan sea salt
  +
- ¼ cup water, room temperature
  +
- ½ cup light agave nectar
- ½ cup cacao powder *(Cacao Barry brand suggested)*
- 5 drops vanilla essence, alcohol-free

Little Chocolate Spheres Instructions

1. Blend first set of ingredients in high-speed blender.
2. Add water and blend again until smooth.
3. Pour into SMALL silicone mold.
   (You might have some extra left. You can keep the remainder of the preparation in refrigerator or freezer for future use [as a white chocolate]) ➤

4. Freeze overnight.

5. Blend last set of ingredients until smooth.

6. Pour into the BROWNIE mold and freeze overnight.

Tempered Chocolate Bomb Ingredients

- 3 cups cacao powder
- 1 cup cacao butter
- ½ cup light agave nectar or coconut nectar
- 15 drops vanilla extract, alcohol-free
- ⅛ tsp Himalayan sea salt

Tempered Chocolate Bomb Instructions

1. Melt the cacao butter using the double boiler method. The double boiler method basically uses two pieces, a large pot that is filled with hot or boiling water and a smaller pot that fits inside and uses the steam from the hot water to heat the ingredient. That way, the ingredient will not burn.

2. Add the cacao powder to glass bowl. Remove cacao butter from double boiler and pour into bowl.

3. Using a spatula, quickly mix the cacao butter and Cacao Barry powder together until the chocolate is tempered, about 108°F (42 °C), and then slowly bring the temperature down to 88°F (31.5 °C) by moving chocolate around in a fluid motion. **The room must be around 68°F (20 °C) or below and humidity no higher than 50%.**

4. After chocolate is tempered, add vanilla extract and salt, then mix.

5. With a chocolate brush, make sure each half sphere is covered all the way up the edges.

6. Repeat the process for all the 6 spheres. Let sit for 5 minutes.

7. Repeat the covering process a second time.

8. Let sit for 5 minutes, then place in the freezer for 15 minutes.

Pumpkin Sauce Ingredients

- ½ cup mangoes, frozen
- ¼ cup pumpkin, softened using the double boiler method
- ¼ cup raw coconut water
- ⅛ tsp pumpkin spice
- 2 Tbsp light agave nectar or coconut nectar
- 2 drops stevia, alcohol-free
- 5 drops vanilla extract, alcohol-free

Pumpkin Sauce Instructions

1. Blend all ingredients in high-speed blender until smooth.

2. Pour into a shallow container and set aside.

Pumpkin Cream Ingredients

- ½ cup macadamia nuts, rinsed
- ½ cup cacao butter
- 1 Tbsp orange juice
- ⅛ tsp Himalayan sea salt
  +
- ⅜ cup filtered water
  +
- ¼ cup pumpkin puree (made using the double boiler method)
- ½ tsp organic cane sugar

Pumpkin Cream Instructions

1. Blend the first four ingredients in a high-speed blender; blend until smooth.
2. Add the water and blend again until fully smooth.
3. Add the last two ingredients and blend again.
4. Pour in a shallow container and set aside. **Do not rinse the blender**.

Citrus Crumble Ingredients

- ¼ cup pumpkin cream
- ¼ cup raspberries, frozen
- ½ cup pumpkin sauce
- ⅛ cup coconut water

Citrus Crumble Instructions

1. Blend for 3 minutes all ingredients in high-speed blender (the previous one that was **not** rinsed off).
2. Pour into a shallow container and set aside.

Decoration Ingredients

- 1 tsp pumpkin pulp
- 1 homegrown mature sprout (or any other seed that gives a green color)
- 2-3 Tbsp raspberry sauce
- ¼ cup raspberries, freeze-dried

ASSEMBLY

1. Pour pumpkin sauce into a white round shape plate.
2. Take ½ bomb and scoop 2-3 Tbsp citrus crumble.
3. Fill to ¾ by placing delicately in the center of the Pumpkin Sauce.
4. Add the freeze dried raspberries.
5. Add a couple of the chocolate spheres, preferably the larger ones from the 9 x 2.75 x 0.9-inch silicone mold.
6. Add the sprout for decoration on the top.
7. Using tweezers, add a little bit of the pumpkin pulp on top of the second half of the chocolate bomb.
8. Serve immediately or refrigerate for up to 7 days. The extra half spheres can be frozen for future use if needed.

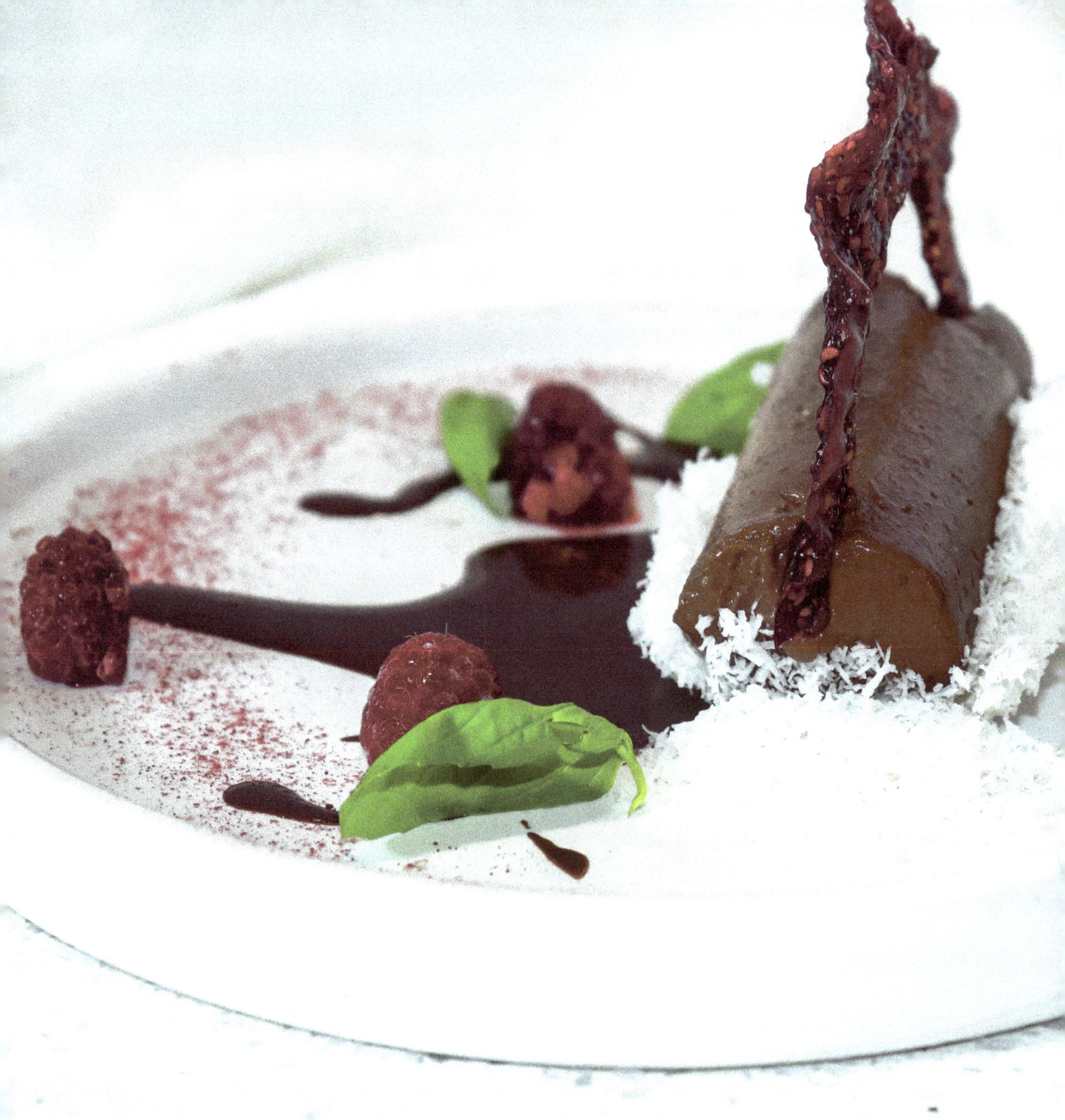

Chocolate Fudge Snow

Serving size: 5 chocolate logs

Equipment

- High-speed blender
- Dehydrator
- Spatula
- Mixing bowl
- 9-Cavity (*brand Silikomart*) Silicone log mold 2.8 oz, 1¼ x 3⁵⁄₁₆ x 1⅜ inches
- Round cookie cutter
- An offset spatula
- Food grade gloves
- White round-shaped plate
- Sift
- Tweezers
- Whisk

Raspberry Arc Ingredients

- ½ cup organic raspberries, thawed
- 2 Tbsp coconut nectar

Raspberry Arc Instructions

1. Add the ingredients for the raspberry arc to a mixing bowl.
2. Using a whisk, bring the mixture to a thick consistency.
3. Line a dehydrator with parchment paper.
4. Pour the mixture on the parchment paper.
5. Dehydrate for about 24 hours.
   Note: The mixture should not be completely dry. We want it a bit soft so it can be cut using the round-shaped cookie cutter.
6. Using the cookie cutter, cut the raspberry to obtain a cylinder shape and dehydrate again for 14 hours
7. Put in the refrigerator for 1 hour to harden a bit.
   Note: The outer part of the cut is what is needed. The inner part can be put in a sealed bag and put in the freezer for future use.
8. Remove from the refrigerator.
9. Gently peel the outer part of the raspberry arc with your hands.
10. Using scissors, cut the cylinder shape of the raspberry into 2 pieces. *(Only one piece will be used for this recipe. The other piece can be stored in the freezer in a sealed container bag for future use.)* ➤

Chocolate Fudge Ingredients

- 2½ cup walnuts, soaked for 4 hours, rinsed and dehydrated
- ⅔ cup coconut nectar
- ½ cup cacao powder, raw
- ½ cup water, filtered
- 8 drops vanilla extract, alcohol-free
- 2 Tbsp juice of an orange
- ⅛ tsp Himalayan sea salt
  +
- ¼ cup melted coconut oil

Chocolate Fudge Instructions

1. Add all the ingredients of the chocolate fudge to a high-speed blender (*except the coconut oil*); blend until combined. (*You might need your spatula or tamper in case the mixture gets stuck and blend again. The mixture might look grainy. It is completely normal.*)
2. Add the coconut oil and blend again for about 10 seconds.
3. Put your silicone mold on a non-wooden tray
4. Pour the chocolate fudge in each cavity until you fill 5 of the cavities.
5. Using your offset spatula, remove any excess fudge on the surface.
6. Tap the tray a couple times to remove any air bubbles.
7. Put in freezer for 8 hours or overnight.

Chocolate Ganache Ingredients

- ½ cup cacao butter
- ¼ cup raw cacao powder
- 2 Tbsp coconut nectar
- 2 drops vanilla extract, alcohol-free

Chocolate Ganache Instructions

1. Melt the cacao butter using the double boiler method.
2. Add the remaining ingredients to the cacao powder.
3. Using a whisk, mix until well combined.

Decoration Ingredients

- 3 raspberries, fresh
- 1 tsp organic dried beet powder
- 1 bouquet mint leaves
- 3 cups fine shredded coconut, unsweetened
- 1 Tbsp organic acerola powder

ASSEMBLY

1. Add 1 tablespoon of the melted chocolate ganache to the round plate and slowly tilt the plate to make a chocolate drip effect (*do not tilt it so much that the drip touches the edge of the bowl*).
2. Refrigerate the remainder of the ganache in a shallow container for future use.
3. Remove the chocolate fudge from the freezer.
4. Using gloves, remove 1 bar. Leave the remaining bars in the freezer for future use. (*You can repurpose them into another recipe.*)
5. Add acerola powder to a sifter and tap gently to pour some of the powder on the chocolate fudge. This will give a slightly shiny appearance to the fudge.
6. Take a mixing bowl and add the shredded coconut to it. Use gloves to hold each end of 1 chocolate bar (from freezer), let the coconut stick to the bottom of the bar.
   Note: At room temperature, the chocolate will start melting quickly so you might move quickly for this process. Remove the bar from the bowl (allowing some of

the coconut to stay on it), and place it on the edge of the chocolate (starting point of the drip effect)

7. Add the dried beet powder to a sift.

8. Release some of the beet powder on the plate by tapping the sift gently with your hand.

9. Using tweezers, add the fresh raspberries sparingly on the plate.

10. Add a mint leaf close to each raspberry.

11. Top the chocolate bar with the raspberry arc.

12. Refrigerate for 5 minutes before serving. This is to allow the chocolate ganache to set.

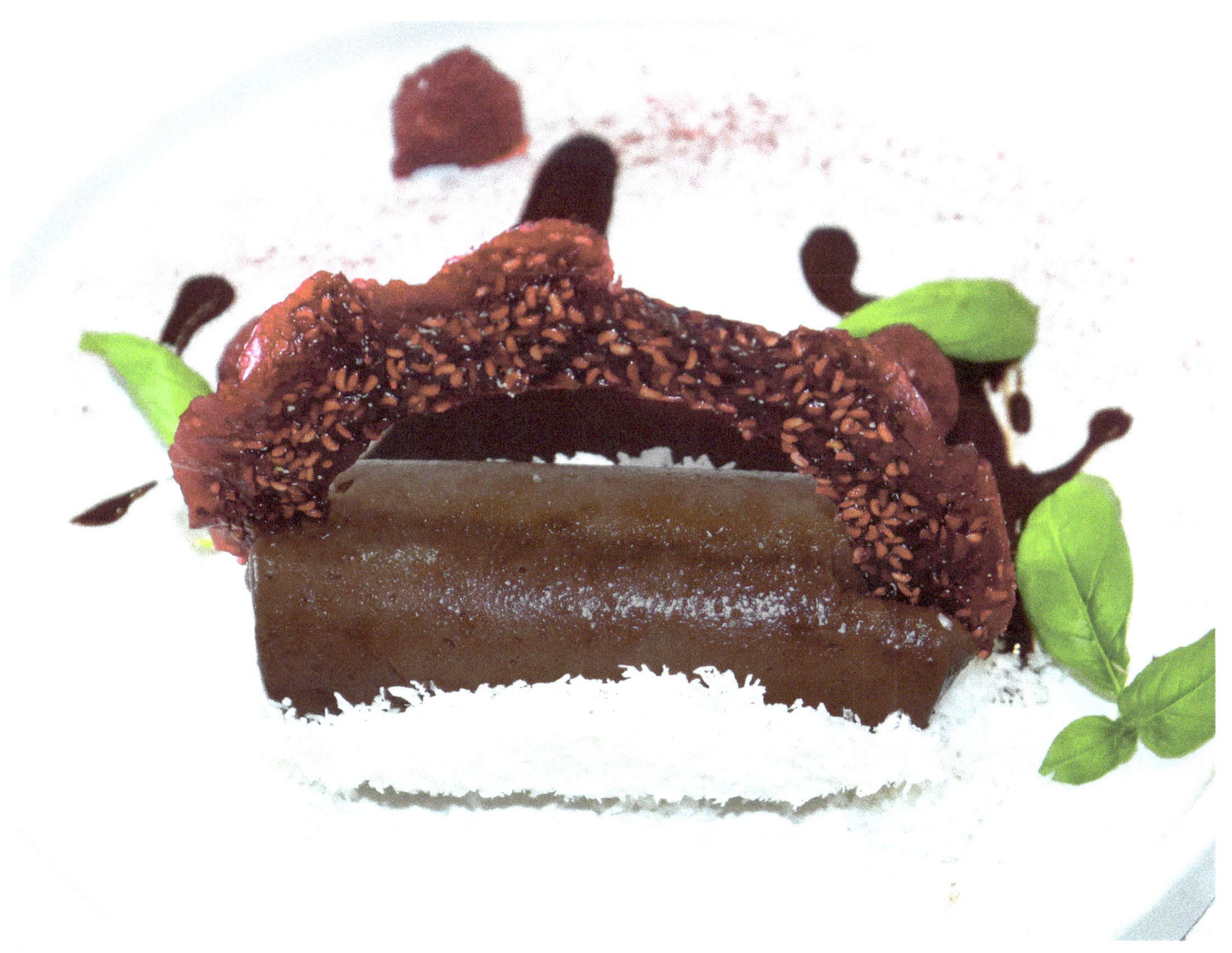

Thank You!

Index